Community As Healing

Community As Healing

Pragmatist Ethics in Medical Encounters

D. Micah Hester

ROWMAN & LITTLEFIELD PUBLISHERS, INC.
Lanham • Boulder • New York • Oxford

ROWMAN & LITTLEFIELD PUBLISHERS, INC.

Published in the United States of America
by Rowman & Littlefield Publishers, Inc.
4720 Boston Way, Lanham, Maryland 20706
www.rowmanlittlefield.com

12 Hid's Copse Road
Cumnor Hill, Oxford OX2 9JJ, England

British Library Cataloguing in Publication Information Available

Library of Congress Cataloging-in-Publication Data

Hester, D. Micah.
  Community as healing : pragmatist ethics in medical encounters / D. Micah Hester.
    p. cm.
  Includes bibliographical references and index.
  ISBN 0-7425-1218-5 (cloth : alk. paper) — ISBN 0-7425-1219-3 (pbk. : alk. paper)
    1. Medical ethics. 2. Medical ethics—Social aspects. I. Title.

R724 .H47 2001
174'.2—dc21

                                                                  00-054437

Printed in the United States of America

∞™ The paper used in this publication meets the minimum requirements of American
National Standard for Information Sciences—Permanence of Paper for Printed Library
Materials, ANSI/NISO Z.39.48-1992.

Contents

Preface

It is often said that you learn as much or more by teaching than by being a student, and this is certainly true in my case. But at no time has this statement applied more acutely than in fall 1993 when, as a new adjunct assistant professor at Tennessee State University, I was given an almost overwhelming task to teach a course I had only passing acquaintance with, a course on medical ethics. Now, most professors at one time or another teach some courses that are new to them for which, one hopes, they take the summer or winter break to prepare carefully their syllabi and so forth. However, in my case, no such luxury was afforded me since I found out I was teaching the course on the first day of the fall semester.

This was, not surprisingly, one of those good news/bad news situations. The good news was that the previous spring I had audited an undergraduate Ethics and Medicine class taught by Richard Zaner of Vanderbilt University; the bad news was that the course was my *only* exposure to this area of study. The other good news was that I did not have to go through the hassle of choosing a textbook; the bad news was that I had 36 hours in which to design a syllabus with no prior knowledge of the textbook or reflection upon the class and its contents.

All of this made for a fascinating semester where I did my best to stay a step ahead of my students, trying primarily to lead discussions on important social issues in medicine. Instead of lecturing, I relied on case studies and the textbook to give substance to the issues, while I asked questions of the students and wrote random words on the board when I thought they were significant. The students found themselves as confused by the whole matter as I was, and I was finding it increasingly difficult to probe the questions raised by the cases using the tools at hand—namely, the textbook. In particular, coming from a background of American pragmatism, where philosophers like William James, John Dewey, and George Herbert Mead stressed that the dichotomies between theory and practice as well as self and community are artificial and problematic, I began to wonder why bioethics was so wrapped up in the so-called "Georgetown mantra" of four "biomedical" principles (autonomy, beneficence, nonmaleficence, and justice) and a supposed adversarial relationship between individuals and society. The articles in the textbook simply had little in the way of either phenomenological or pragmatic discussions of ethical issues in medicine.

So I began to look to other textbooks, a few monographs, journal articles, and so forth, and what I found was that (save for a few strong but relatively ignored voices) American pragmatism had little say in the field of bioethics. Certainly, in the "mainstream" discussions and within the professional societies of the time, pragmatism was virtually nonexistent as a method for handling bioethical issues. These facts, as I saw them then, led me to begin my own research in the field, and no aspect of bioethics seemed (or seems) to me more central than issues covered under the broad topic known as "physician–patient relationships" or "medical encounters." It is in the interaction between health care professional and laypatient that "the rubber hits the road," as it were. Ethical issues are social issues; the actions of individuals often profoundly affect others around them. Clearly, this is the case in medicine, and yet the "theoretical" attempts of bioethicists to resolve conflicts rarely hit their mark.

The following text is an attempt to rethink or reconstruct medical encounters from the standpoint of classic American pragmatism. The argument begins in chapter 1 with a broad overview of the project, primarily laying out the structure, though surely not the full content, of the argument. Chapter 2 critiques two well-known (if not, admittedly, overcritiqued) forces in contemporary bioethics, Tom Beauchamp/James Childress and H. Tristram Engelhardt, suggesting that the arguments they develop give us vacuous principles that are in practice useless for moral medicine. Chapter 3 then turns to the specific principle of autonomy championed by these authors, arguing that it ultimately leaves us with an empty notion of the self. Chapter 4 then sets forth my positive account of the self as a situated social product, à la Dewey and Mead. Finally, chapter 5 shows how my reconstructed notion of the self can be used to help gain insight into issues of bioethics for medical encounters.

The entire project is guided by the following normative concept: Bioethics should attempt to help patients (as well as physicians and other health care professionals, family, and friends) live significant, meaningful lives at least while they are patients and, hopefully, beyond.

Acknowledgments

Permit me to take a moment (and a few pages) to acknowledge those who have made a difference to my life and this work. Though I take sole responsibility for the positions expressed and the resulting errors in structure and content, this book is the result of a community effort; how could it be otherwise?

I want to begin by paying my respects to my two strongest academic influences, Professors Michael Hodges and John Lachs. Hodges deserves the most credit for getting me through the initial stages of this project (a dissertation, now highly revised). His great sympathy for Dewey and his careful reading and rereading of my original work *made* it happen, and his encouragement all along the way kept it rather painless. He is both an effective editor and a gracious advisor while always being a very good friend. Meanwhile, Lachs's generosity with his time and energy along with his vast knowledge of American philosophy cannot be overpraised. I am simply in awe of a man so thoroughly engaged in the work and profession of philosophy who, at the same time, gives so much of himself to his students and friends.

Of course, I was also quite fortunate to have had an insightful advisor on matters of medicine and ethics, Professor Richard Zaner. Along with his colleagues, Stuart Finder and Mark Bliton in the Vanderbilt University Medical Center's Center for Clinical and Research Ethics, Zaner has given his time and energy to consult with me about philosophy and medicine, time that has been valuable to my understanding of the enterprise in which I am now thoroughly immersed.

Keeping me honest in my approach to the institution of medicine, Robert La-Grone, M.D., spent countless hours listening to me drone on about American pragmatism, *under*educating him in ways too numerous to mention. On the other hand, I have been enlightened greatly by his comments and insights.

Others who deserve mention are Professors James Montmarquet and William Hardy at Tennessee State University, both of whom helped me start my teaching career and encouraged me as I went along. Professors Glenn McGee and Patrick

Shade aided me in developing a better understanding of medical ethics and pragmatism. Robert Talisse (City University of New York, Hunter College) along with Professors Mary Mahowald (University of Chicago), Jonathan Moreno (University of Virginia Medical Center), and John Arras (University of Virginia) have each read portions of chapters, in previous incarnations, that have led to the current look, feel, and content of the work. I also wish to thank the Society for the Advancement of American Philosophy and the Society for Health and Human Values, at which I read papers that have been folded into this work. Furthermore, portions of the following arguments have been expressed in an article in the *Journal of Medicine and Philosophy* (see Hester 1998, and chapter 5) as well as in the anthology from Vanderbilt University Press entitled *Pragmatic Bioethics*, edited by Glenn McGee (see McGee 1999, Hester 1999, and chapters 1 and 5).

A special note of thanks needs to be passed along to Professor John J. McDermott at Texas A&M University. He suggested the notion of "community as healing," which is the central theme of this work. Furthermore, John is a thoroughly engaged self who supports his colleagues with energy and enthusiasm. I am one of the many who considers John as both a teacher and a friend.

My own institution, Mercer University's School of Medicine, deserves special notice, not only for employing me in this fascinating field of bioethics, but also for providing me the time and space to work on this manuscript. In this respect, Dean Robert J. Moon, my direct boss, and Earnestine Waters, my secretary, deserve a special thank-you.

Of course, I cannot leave out the special care and interest with which the publisher, Rowman & Littlefield, has approached this project. Several persons helped bring this work to press, culminating with current philosophy editor, Eve DeVaro.

My decision to go into philosophy/bioethics as a profession was not an easy one. I had a comfortable computer-based job in a beautiful area of the country with good friends nearby. The decision was made easier, however, by the support (albeit with reservations) of my father, James D. Hester (who teaches me the value and limitations of reflection and loyalty), and mother, Darilyn J. Hester (who encourages me to be part of a community and showed me what it means to love), as well as my brother, J. David Hester (who has always taken steps ahead of me that have helped me find my own path).

Finally, the good fortunes that have befallen me during this entire enterprise are no better exemplified than by the great luck that came my way during my time in graduate school when I met my wife, Kelly Sherman(-Hester). She has put up with my antics and relocations for many years now, an imprisonment I would never wish on anyone, but she has found ways to push through with me. Her love and support have been invaluable, incalculable, and incredible. For not only this, but also for giving us and raising our beautiful daughter Emily, all *my* love *and* the dedication of this work go to her.

Abbreviations

Throughout this work, I use the author-date text-citation format as described in *The Chicago Manual of Style*, 14th ed. (1993), with the following exceptions here noted (see references in this book for complete information):

FB [year] for Engelhardt Jr., H. Tristram. 1986. *The Foundations of Bioethics.* New York: Oxford University Press.

——. 1996. *The Foundations of Bioethics.* 2d ed. New York: Oxford University Press.

PBE [year] for Beauchamp, Tom, and James Childress. 1979. *Principles of Biomedical Ethics.* New York: Oxford University Press.

——. 1994. *Principles of Biomedical Ethics.* 4th ed. New York: Oxford University Press.

References to the critical editions of John Dewey are abbreviated using initials for the series and the number of the volume in the following form: series/volume, page number(s). For example, a reference to *Theory of Valuation*, vol. 13, *The Later Works*, page 220, would be abbreviated (LW13, 220).

Chapter 1

Medicine, Ethics, and Classic American Philosophy

Each decade since the mid-1950s has seen an increase in the number of treatises produced in the emerging field of bioethics. Particularly in the past decade, the number of individuals involved in the thought processes and practices of bioethics grew at an almost exponential rate. At the same time hundreds, even thousands of articles, journals, books, Internet sites, and television broadcasts have been dedicated to topics in bioethics by professionals in medicine, law, and clinical ethics. Have we hit saturation?

Of course, it is important to recognize that contemporary bioethics has developed in direct response to a twentieth-century trend in medicine toward technological solutions, coercive paternalism, and invasive disease eradication.[1] A world at war in the first half of the twentieth century led to a heightened sense of urgency in medicine to find miracle cures for disease and bodily destruction. An *ethos* in medicine was cultivated that developed the "research" paradigm as the goal of good medicine. Disease became the focus of medical practice such that patients found little room in which to interact with physicians. They were regarded as complexes of microscopic biophysical mechanisms that develop and combat disease rather than as active, participating agents in the healing process.[2] Human experimentation was, and is, widely performed, raising the question of whom to recruit as subjects of experiments and how they should be recruited. In a narrow, utilitarian way, underprivileged and compromised people and groups were targeted; prisoners, women, children, minority ethnic groups, and institutionalized individuals became the pool from which to draw. This heightened emphasis on experimentation and the creation of new, invasive technologies (like new surgical techniques, dialysis machines, etc.) coupled with the already prevailing paternalistic practices of physicians—that is, the attitude that the physician "knows what is best" for the patient—led to the development of acute ethical conflicts that demanded attention.

World War II produced many successful research projects into life-sustaining treatments. Public response to discoveries such as penicillin helped fuel the fire of medical experimentation. However, with the well-publicized Nuremberg trials after World War II, the world of medicine was opened to public scrutiny as we slowly began to realize that research is neither ethically neutral nor always good in itself. Though there was no direct connection between medical research in America and Nazi practices, this public scrutiny soon began to focus attention on conflicts between medical means and ends in the United States as well. The first to respond in academic circles to questionable practices of medicine were theologians of Christian ethics. Figures like Joseph Fletcher and, later, Paul Ramsey began to request that the "personhood" of the patient not be lost in the technological workings of medicine, that medicine attempt to view its practices from the patient's point of view.[3] However, it was not until the mid-1960s, when medical practitioners themselves started to question the activities of medicine, that bioethics truly began to take shape as an academic discipline.[4]

The decade of the 1960s brought the advent of new medical technologies—for example, ultrasonography, home dialysis, computer-aided therapy, and transplantation. Physicians now had at their disposal highly sophisticated knowledge and abilities that could save and improve lives that only a decade before would have been lost. These abilities often seemed miraculous and led to a heightened enthusiasm for medical science and progress. However, these "miracles" of science also had their controversial sides. For example, the availability of expensive and limited renal dialysis in the early 1960s led to the controversial rationing scheme of a Seattle kidney institute where a committee mostly of "laypeople" developed conditions to be met in order for a patient to receive dialysis. These conditions were, in part, social "judgments" concerning candidates based on perceived ties and contributions to society under the guise that they had "found a fairly reasonable and simple solution to an impossibly difficult problem" (Belding Scribner, quoted in Pence 2000, 324). In another case, Dr. Christiaan Barnard's first "successful" heart transplant into patient Louis Washkansky raised questions of egoism when the media frenzy surrounding the surgery lost sight of the patient, focusing on the "accomplishments of the 44-year-old South African surgeon." This is strikingly problematic given that the patient lived for only eighteen days after surgery—about five of which are reported to have been "very good, happy days" (Pence 2000, 284).[5]

The early and middle part of the following decade brought little relief to the arena of bioethical discussion. Further revelations of unethical practices came with the news of the Tuskegee study in which it was discovered that 399 men with late-stage syphilis went untreated for the duration of a U.S. Public Health experiment that lasted forty years (1932–72), continuing more than thirty years after the discovery and manufacturing of a known cure, penicillin (Jones 1993; Reverby 2000; Pence 1995, 225–52). And a few years later, the now (in)famous legal battle over the plight of a permanent vegetative state (PVS) patient, Karen

Ann Quinlan (1975–76) captured headlines when the family of the 21-year-old woman was blocked in its attempt to remove life-support technologies.[6]

During these times, bioethics was still a very new field and was yet to have a strong response to the ever-changing landscape of medicine.

All this changed, however, in the late 1970s when a landmark work by Tom Beauchamp and James Childress, *Principles of Biomedical Ethics*, was published. As a reaction to controversies in medical practice, Beauchamp and Childress offered a method of ethical inquiry that applies basic bioethical principles to problematic ethical situations in medicine. As I will discuss in chapter 2, their book places a priority on four principles that are supposed to delimit clearly the ethical playing field in medicine. These four principles are (respect for) autonomy, beneficence, nonmaleficence, and justice. The principle of autonomy in particular (discussed in chapter 3) is championed as most important among these principles and is expressed both in a negative form as the need to provide an absence of coercive influences on a patient's decision-making process and in a positive yet passive form as "*express* and informed consent" (PBE 1994, 128).

A few years later in the mid-1980s, H. Tristram Engelhardt published another seminal text in bioethics entitled *The Foundations of Bioethics*. As I will also explain in chapter 2, Engelhardt takes an approach to ethics that leads him to promote two principles of bioethics: the principle of autonomy (permission) and the principle of beneficence. Like Immanuel Kant's concept of autonomy, Engelhardt's principle, in particular, is formal, described as the necessary condition for the possibility of morality. Though of different philosophical origin from Beauchamp/Childress, oddly enough Engelhardt, too, reduces the principle of autonomy (again, chapter 3) in practical situations to the demand for "free consent of those involved" (FB 1986, 85).

In subsequent years, the respective positions taken by Beauchamp/Childress and Engelhardt have developed a strong following within the disciplines of both bioethics and medicine. Noticeably among the practitioners of medicine, the "ethical" vocabulary of "autonomy" and "beneficence" is frequently employed. Physicians and nurses alike attempt to justify their actions toward patients either by way of "consent" or as being in their patients' "best interest." Autonomy itself is championed as the basic right of every patient (though this right is frequently ignored), and formal procedures have been developed specifically around the idea of autonomy and are manifested in such items as "informed consent" forms and "patients' rights" documents.[7] Ultimately, however, the principle of autonomy as exemplified by these authors has no active ("positive") response to coercion; that is, they contain no promotion of agency and participation in medical decisions. Patients are not empowered by the principle of autonomy; they are merely protected. Patients are not made participants in their own treatment but are only shielded from blatant forms of unconsented-to activity by health care professionals. No useful instruments of agency are developed through the "application" of the principle of autonomy, which is a fundamental reason why it falls short as a basis for biomedical ethics.

Both in response to these and other inadequacies and in an attempt to bring a greater diversity of philosophical insights to bear on medicine, several bioethicists have developed theories based on virtue ethics (Pellegrino and Thomasma 1993; Shelp 1985), casuistry (Jonsen and Toulmin 1988; Jonsen, Siegler, and Winslade 1992), rules (Clouser and Gert 1990; Gert 1988), contract-partnership models (Veatch 1981, 1991), and care (Blustein 1991), among others. Today, a large variety of bioethics titles line the shelves of medical libraries. Seemingly all camps are now being heard from, and many viable solutions to problems in medical encounters exist on those shelves. So, even if Beauchamp/Childress and Engelhardt fall short, surely others have written something to carry us forth. And if not, still others claim that writing may not matter anyway since the "real" work of bioethics does not and cannot go on in the pages of books but in the clinic, at the bedside. Thus, we must ask a significant question: *Why another treatise on the subject?* Perhaps the pages of this work will speak for themselves. However, let me attempt to begin the answer here directly.

Poring over the literature in the field of bioethics, one sees that many philosophical camps have spoken. Utilitarian, deontological, and virtue theorists all have their say, though some more frequently and more loudly than others. Surprisingly, however, in a discipline developed primarily in response not simply to the general medical practices of the West but to specific medical encounters in the United States, authors who write in a classical American vein—writers in the tradition of C. S. Peirce, William James, John Dewey, and George Herbert Mead (to name but a few)—have been given little voice. Rarely do you find medical ethics anthologies with American pragmatist or naturalist essays, and even more rarely do professional discussions occur using the conceptions and vocabulary of American pragmatism.[8]

I contend that this missing (or, at least, sparingly heard) voice in bioethics is highly regrettable, and the pages that follow attempt to give an account of a pragmatist's perspective that may help right this wrong by bringing the thoughts of classical American authors to bear on medical encounters between patients and health care professionals. The pragmatist tradition, it seems to me, is uniquely suited to approach contemporary ethical issues since pragmatists have always emphasized the integration of theory and practice and the relevance of philosophy to living. With a focus on the method and activity of inquiry, the importance of rational and affective dimensions in reflective thought, and the integration of means and ends, individuals and community, pragmatism provides a unique, rich, and positive "theory" of ethics that can enlighten encounters among individuals. Further, pragmatism has always been suspicious of sharp dichotomies like mind/body, individual/society, and, for that matter, physician/patient, dichotomies that saturate the field of bioethics.

Pragmatism brings to the bioethical table a vast array of rich resources—resources that have great affinities with other bioethical movements like virtue, narrative, and feminist ethics. I wish to take advantage of these resources by focusing attention on medicine and medical encounters. In particular, I will attempt to reconceive physician–patient relationships in light of a *pragmatic understanding of moral intelligence and artistry performed by socially situated selves that develop into and arise out of an attitude of community as healing*. It is the brief "unpacking" of this dense statement to which I turn for the remainder of this chapter and which sets out the issues to be developed throughout the rest of this book.

PRAGMATIC UNDERSTANDING: INTELLIGENT HABITS AND HABITS OF INTELLIGENCE[9]

Just in the degree in which a physician is an artist in his work he uses his science, no matter how extensive and accurate, to furnish him with tools of inquiry into the individual case, and with methods of forecasting a method of dealing with it. Just in the degree in which, no matter how great his learning, he subordinates the individual case to some classification of diseases and some generic rule of treatment, he sinks to the level of the routine mechanic. His intelligence and his action become rigid, dogmatic, instead of free and flexible. (MW12, 176)

Practice of any sort is a function of habits, and the activities and attitudes of medical practitioners are no exception.[10] Habits of medicine are quite pronounced (from history-taking to routine blood pressure checks); of particular concern are those habits of physicians that have stagnated, that make "intelligence . . . and action . . . rigid, dogmatic, instead of free and flexible." These habits I will generally term "habituations." Dogmatic physicians—that is, physicians who function out of habituation—miss the fact that as part of the environment in which the physician operates, differences among patients require sensitive adjudication by the physician in order to foster successful encounters. As physician/philosopher Edmund Pellegrino has pointed out, physicians who practice by rote run the risk of developing poor clinical/medical judgments while they ignore the desires and interests of their patients as unique individuals as well.

Pellegrino, echoing Dewey's warning against the subordination of the individual case to generic disease classifications, argues that the end of a medical encounter is "a right healing action for *a particular patient*" (Pellegrino 1979, 173 [emphasis mine]). His continuing emphasis on the particularity of the patient translates to a decisive move away from basic "textbook" investigation of symptoms and biological processes, which if left unchecked by and unintegrated with the larger social aspects of the individuals in the situation—aspects that make the patient unique—provides the environment for clinical judgments to suffer and runs the risk of missing the desired ends of the medical encounter. Each patient brings to the table a new situation never before encountered. Though at times symptoms and conditions are usefully and necessarily classifiable into previously known categories, these general notions of disease are never merely ends in themselves but are instrumental means of questioning and investigating that eventuate in a *specific* "right healing action." Medicine, therefore, can never merely be a strict science of classification but an art form that imaginatively applies the instruments of medical science based on careful investigation, dialectic, probability, and communication. In order to heal *this patient*, "[d]ecisive action frequently involves the counterposition of what is good scientifically, what the physician *thinks* is good, and what the patient will accept as good" (Pellegrino 1979, 180). Thus, "[i]n making the 'right' decision for an individual patient . . . personal, social, economic, and psychological characteristics of the patient must be factored in" (Pellegrino 1979, 181). Intelligent solutions require attention to the individual case, and clinical practice, in its attempt to bring about a healthy patient, is no less immune to the dangers of rote, dogmatic practice, than is any other occupation. Not simply bad personal interaction but *bad medicine* results from inattention to the differences and uniqueness of each case, each particular patient. "Medicine must not only perform well but act well, it must choose what should be done to heal a particular patient whose good is the true end of the whole activity" (Pellegrino 1979, 191).

It is clear, then, that both Dewey and Pellegrino would agree that "dogmatic" physicians are in danger of practicing bad medicine in a world where "good" medicine necessarily involves a whole complex of issues related to biochemistry, sociology, psychology, and ethics. Habits in their dogmatic application act efficiently but rigidly, whether they are diagnostic or therapeutic; they do not treat the particular patient but a general "type." Individuality of the patient is lost since that individuality is not found in "textbook" cases but in the social and cultural aspects of the people involved in the situation; individuals are created and discovered in relation to others—that is, to communities. Science in its "pure" form relies on general principles, and "scientific" medicine is no exception. But art is individual; it is unique. And medicine as an art form must investigate and treat the individual patient, not a general type.

What can be done about this? How might we counteract those "dogmatic" habits of physicians so much a part of the culture in which they find themselves? I suggest that the "science" of medicine, in order to become an "art form," would benefit, at least in part, from an infusion of intelligent habits of community that treat patients, in their unique individuality, as *members* of the health care community.

It may help us, then, to understand what is meant here by "habit." Habits are controlled adjustments of individual *and* environment that are at ready disposal within a given situation. They are tendencies to act, tendencies that have been acquired. Note that the breadth of this definition entails that habits can be found anywhere humans reside, infused in anything of human character.[11] We readily accept that many of our physical actions are habits, but beyond this, Peirce, James, and Dewey have shown us that beliefs are habits, emotions are habits, and even ideas are habits (cf. Peirce 1992; James [1890] 1950; and MW14).[12] For example, the recognition that the back window of my car has been broken motivates blood flow to my face, a look at my watch, a realization that some of the electronics in the car are gone, and a brisk movement back toward the house while talking to myself about my misfortune. These activities constitute my idea that something is wrong, my belief that I am the victim of some crime, and my emotional frustration and worry.

But further, these activities occur as functions of habits, as actions waiting in reserve mobilized by the circumstances in which I find myself. (Violation of property sets in motion my habits of fear, frustration, investigation, and stress.) As American pragmatists have pointed out, what we call ideas, beliefs, and emotions are general terms applied to biological and cultural habits after these habits have been investigated. We do not believe or emote first, then act. The act is the belief or emotion. Habits are stimulated, and we perform.

However, this may sound as if habits control our activities to the extent that we cannot be said to act intelligently but automatically according to the direction of our habits. Nothing could be further from the truth. Habits and intelligence relate in a number of, admittedly paradoxical, ways.

> Habits are a condition of intellectual efficiency. They operate in two ways upon intellect. Obviously, they restrict its reach, they fix its boundaries. . . . All habit-forming involves the beginning of an intellectual speculation which if unchecked ends in thoughtless action. . . . Habit is however more than a restriction of thought. Habits become negative limits because they are first positive agencies. The more numerous our habits the wider the field of possible observation and foretelling. The more flexible they are, the more refined is perception in its discrimination and the more delicate the presentation evoked by imagination. (MW14, 121–23)

Dewey contrasts habits unchecked by intelligence (for which they were initially placed into service) with flexible, productive habits that expand intellectual horizons. I wish to call these productive habits "intelligent" insofar as they serve both in means and ends as thoughtful and flexible adjustings of old habits to the uniqueness of each new situation.

> We are always possessed by habits and customs, and this fact signifies that we are always influenced by the inertia and the momentum of forces temporarily outgrown but nevertheless still present with us as a part of our being. . . . [However, i]n its largest sense . . . remaking of the old through union with the new is precisely what intelligence is. (LW11, 36–37)

Opposed to these productive, intelligent habits, there are those habits that, though they may provide a kind of efficiency in action, end in thoughtless routine that stifles rather than promotes further intelligent activity. I call these thoughtless habits "habituations." They take the environment (at the time) as fixed and uniform; thus, "adjustment is just fitting ourselves to this fixity of external conditions" (MW9, 51). Habituations are mechanical and routine. Whereas habits in their fullest sense are readily reflected upon (even if only in small ways), habituations are habit-developed activities that are performed in a relatively unreflective manner. To quote Dewey again,

> Habit as *habituation* is indeed something *relatively* passive. . . . Conformity to the environment, a change wrought in the organism without reference to ability to modify surroundings, is a marked trait of . . . habituations. . . . Habituation is [in part] . . . *our adjustment to an environment which at the time we are not concerned with modifying.* (MW9, 51–52 [emphasis mine])

An example to clarify the differences might be in order here.

Most mornings a large segment of the adult population of the United States shaves some part of the body. The ritual is common, but not without its nicks and scratches. When we first learn to shave, the experience is awkward. We fear the blade and are tentative with each scrape and around every curve. However, as the number of our experiences increases and occurs with greater regularity, our fears subside; tentative movements give way to confident flourishes. Simply approaching the razor begins within us a mobilization of forces. Seeing the gleaming blade, reaching for the shave cream launches our muscles and thoughts into a customized routine. This is the expression of a multiplicity of habits in all their great tendencies toward action. However, reflection is usually not lost. The least-wounded shavers continue to be aware of the nuances of the face or legs or whatever. They recognize blemishes that must be handled with care, bones that must be traversed with greater sensitivity than loose flesh. Subtle habits are mobilized, gripping the blade firmly but deftly, adjusting that grip along the way, stretching and contorting the face. We are all aware of the unreflective times, however. Those times of pure habituation that often result in cuts—the careless twist of the handle slicing an edge across the skin, the unthinking scrape that digs a bit too deep, presses a bit too hard, the use of blades too dull to cut hair at all. We take the situation to be so "routine" that our activities function on "automatic pilot," and yet we soon curse our own stupidity while reaching for something to stop the bleeding.

Do not be seduced by the simplicity of this example. It depicts a familiar scene where the habits are covert, the necessary reflection is quick, the adjustments between organism and environment are minuscule. Furthermore, its familiarity and its connection to bodily movement may obscure my point, for as we have seen above, habits function mentally as well as physically. Bodily habits—shaving, walking, eating—are those we experience primarily from the perspective of their physical aspects, while others—thinking, dreaming, emoting—(and yes, these are habits, or functions thereof) may be taken from the perspective of their so-called mental aspects. Without going too deeply into pragmatic and functional epistemology and psychology, suffice it to say that thoughts and emotions well up inside us as responses to our environment, responses that are available to us primarily from our storehouse of socialized habits of thinking and feeling. They are the results of "physical" changes and adaptations as much as they are forms of "mental" gymnastics or "private" affections (cf. James [1890] 1950).[13] Dewey explains this well: "The significance of habit is not exhausted . . . in its executive and motor phase. It means formation of intellectual and emotional disposition as well as an increase in ease, economy, and efficiency of action" (MW9, 52–53). Again, let me elucidate by way of example.

On the day that I am writing this, the clouds are out, the temperature is cool, the climate is rainy, and, to top it off, it is Monday. As I investigate my mood, I find that I lack energy, my job is distasteful, people annoy me; that is, I am generally depressed (not "clinically," I hope). Depression is an emotion or psychological state of, as we might commonly say, "feeling down." When depressed, pessimism guides future concerns, and little can be done to cheer one up. That describes my state as I write this. But why am I in such a mood; what are its causes? I suggest that this depression is a function of habits, habits brought on by my environment and the way I have become accustomed to dealing with the circumstances of days like today. And surely many people have had similar experiences. Quite simply I have "programmed" myself into depression on most rainy days. Couple this with the realization that it is the first day of a new workweek, and a pool of responsive habits are put into play to bring me down. Certainly, this explanation is viable, but one thing that makes it interesting is that we are not focusing on overtly physical aspects of life. These habits are primarily what we call emotive, psychological, and mental. Thus, we have stretched the "ordinary" reach of habits into the fuller force of life, in both its mental and physical arenas.

Habits, however, are, in the words of Donald Morris, a "double-edged sword." As Morris points out, "By forming habits we restrict the need for conscious consideration of what we are doing. As a result our thoughts are bounded by specific limits, and we may fail to consider all possibilities" (Morris 1996, 38). Dewey says, "A habit marks an *inclination*—an active preference and choice for the conditions involved in its exercise" (MW9, 53). As "inclinations," habits "prefer" and "choose" the conditions that call them forth; they do not passively wait in reserve but seek out conditions in which to act. They attempt, at least upon first appearance, to be exercised in particular ways along very restricted lines. The active nature of habits can lead to the "unthinking" exercise of them. Again, from Dewey:

> Routine habits are unthinking habits. . . . [T]he acquiring of habits is due to an original plasticity of our natures: to our ability to vary responses till we find an appropriate and efficient way of acting. Routine habits, and habits that possess us instead of our possessing them, are habits which put an end to plasticity. They mark the close of power to vary. (MW9, 54)

These routine habits that I have termed habituations are the dangerous side of habits since they lose the ability to be exercised intelligently. Their "rote" nature makes them incapable of working (except by accident) for the benefit of any situation since each new situation is going to require some variation in our habits. To disrupt these patterns takes other habits, habits of reflection and deliberation that need to be activated in order to check habits before they become habituations.

Habits of shaving are efficient yet dangerous if we are not attentive to the present environment. Habits of depression are acceptable in moderation but pathological if they control moods without restriction. Thus, in order to develop intelligent habits—that is, flexible, adaptive, productive habits—we must first cultivate habits of intelligence.

Intelligence is a complex of habits that work together to produce reflective thought and action. These habits include suspending judgment, deliberation, experimentation, and mostly the courage to act checked by an acceptance of fallibility. And each of these habits can be broken into still further detailed habits. Suspended judgments rely on habits of patience and prudence. Deliberation takes imagination in the form of dramatic reconstructions of the situation. Experimentation needs habits that help acquire tools as well as determine and order their uses in the situation. Finally, as Dewey says, "The primary prerequisite of critical ability [and activity] is courage. . . . [For] the easy course is always to accept what is handed out" (LW5, 134). Critical reflection requires habits of courage in order to risk enacting intelligent deliberate judgments that may simply be wrong. All these habits of reflective thinking—that is, intelligence (also known as habits of inquiry or pragmatic logic)—embody an imaginative process that helps make otherwise restricted habits flexible and expansive.

Turning back to medicine, then, the practices and attitudes of medical professionals are no less functions of habits than any others. Not only do habits undergird medical practices, but the attitudes and activities of most medical personnel are, unfortunately, more often the function of habituations—that is, unreflective approaches to patient care that run on virtually unchecked—than they are functions of intelligent, reflective habits. From the expectations of physicians about their patients (and vice versa) to taking histories to using a stethoscope or palpating the abdomen, habits of medical practice make encounters with patients efficient but dangerous, possibly stifling positive, flexible interactions with unique individuals and situations.

Of course, this general critique is not unique to medicine. Ethics professors, among others, can also be guilty of simply "going through the paces"; however, in medicine, two important factors make this problem more acute, pervasive, and problematic. First, medicine often comes into play when someone is concerned about her health, and health is typically felt in intimate and sometimes even mortal/vital ways when in the midst of illness or injury. A cough may not simply mean a cold; it could spell pneumonia. A fast heartbeat could be the sign of overexertion or critical heart problems. Patients come to physicians precisely because they *sense* these different possibilities even if they do not *know* them all. (Though academicians may wish that their students experienced education in similar, vital ways, typically they do not.)

Second, the institutions of medicine (from medical education to medical centers to medical insurance to HMOs) provide an environment in which habituations not only thrive but are even encouraged. (Academics, at least at most large comprehensive universities, have not yet been forced to deal with formularies—well, not in most cases. Academic freedom still insulates most instructors from demands by others that costs be cut, only specific material be provided, etc. [I realize that in some ways the days may be numbered here.]) For example, Columbia/HCA, the nation's largest for-profit HMO, during the past decade defined its own business practices primarily in terms of monetary efficiency, not in terms of helping patients.[14] One HMO term for time spent with patients is "medical-loss ratio" (Anders 1996), meaning that the medical encounter is to count as a loss from the standpoint of the "business" of medicine. In turn, demands are placed on health care professionals that time spent with patients be quick and efficient in order to meet the "bottom line." Of course, this does not bode well for intelligent habits that, admittedly, can be more time consuming than simple habituations. Clearly, the environment that the institution of medicine is developing into works against intelligent habits and for habituations.[15]

The danger of any form of habituation is that it turns the practitioner into an automaton, a machine in both action and attitude. For instance, the prevalence of this in medicine is what gives rise to the idea that computer software can be developed to substitute its diagnostic decision making for that of physicians. Medical diagnostic applications like INTERNIST and CADUCEUS from the University of Pittsburgh were developed in the 1980s for just such purposes, and the development of similar programs continues.[16] Simply place certain vital statistics and symptoms into the formula, and a flowchart maps the course of care.[17]

But equal to, if not more problematic than, turning the practitioner into a mechanical object is the fact that the habituations of the practitioner translate into treating the patient as a machine also, or at least a formula-ized member of a standardized grouping—that is, a nonindividual, ignoring the unique content of a patient's life story. Without reflection in activity, medical personnel cannot account for the subtle but important differences among individual patients.

I do not deny that this may work for some encounters; that is, there are relatively "straightforward" occasions when neither party feels misunderstood or unsuccessful in reaching her goals. Stitching up a cut, dealing with the flu, or even setting a broken bone can be, depending on the pervasive level of disruption in a patient's life, occasions where rote practice can work to all parties' satisfaction. But danger lies even in these so-called simple cases, where underlying issues can develop into ongoing or future health problems that may be missed. And as cases get more complex—for example, head injury, cancer, genetic disorders, AIDS, and so forth—the chances of missing the boat both ethically and medically (if these two can be cleanly separated) increase if reflective care is not given.

To return then to Pellegrino, "Medicine exists as medicine only when it engages in the *full range of activities* which constitute clinical judgment and which lead to decisive action in the interest of a *particular* patient" (Pellegrino 1979, 190 [emphasis mine]). Medicine requires "the full range of activities"—that is, reflection, deliberation, and imagination. More to the point, medicine must develop a pragmatic understanding, or habits of intelligence, employed in the service of individual patients as they present themselves and interact in their "personal, social, economic, and psychological characteristics" (Pellegrino 1979, 181). In other words, medicine must rely on artistic methods that recognize the individuality of patients, an individuality that is developed out of the communities of which they are a part.

It is clear that this is a moral issue of the first order, for we are talking about how people relate to each other. These issues concern the treatment of others and the responsibility for that treatment. It is important, then, to inquire into not only the issue of habituation in practice but, further still, what kinds of habits should be developed and perpetuated in medicine in order to fashion moral encounters between medical professionals and patients. The following chapters do just this by exploring the still prevailing account of moral activity in medicine and how that account fails to provide adequate support for empowering physician–patient encounters with the tools necessary for a truly moral interaction. Rather than basing an account of moral rationality on principles and rules (criticized in chapters 2 and 3), I put forth an ethic based on imaginative, intelligent habits—namely, the notion of "moral artistry."

MORAL ARTISTRY

Problem solving is often seen in a formal light—that is, it is taken as mechanical and routine, following specific, repeatable steps. Ethical investigation, too, has been described as the routine application of imperatives or principles, the following of rules and order. But, in fact, much imaginative activity is involved that is simply not captured by mechanical accounts of intelligence. As we noted above with the distinction between and discussion of habits and habituations, *rigid* routine has little place in intelligent activity. Moral deliberation, itself, cannot be rote application of principles and rules; it must be creatively flexible and adaptive.

Recognizing these facts, Steven A. Fesmire argues that moral rationality is best understood through Dewey's concept of dramatic rehearsal. Fesmire emphasizes Dewey's focus on:

> our capacity for *imagination.* Imagination, like *drama,* is story-structured and is spurred by conflicts and contrasts among characters and contingent events. . . . Rather than being a lyric outburst, imagination (and thus the aesthetic) is constrained and guided by the exigencies and pressures of a situation along with our vast array of internalized *social habits.* (Fesmire 1995, 569–70)

As Dewey himself says, "deliberation is a dramatic rehearsal (in imagination) of various compelling possible lines of action" (MW14, 132).

The imagination, then, has a moral function since "[i]n language and imagination *we rehearse the response of others* just as we dramatically enact other consequences" (MW14, 216 [emphasis mine]). This "story-structured" capacity "guided by" environmental pressures, cultural institutions, and social habits helps us deliberate among a variety of ends-in-view in order to choose a particular path to follow. "For deliberation to be brought to a dramatic resolution, it must develop so as to have a form that expresses coherently the conflicts that originally set the problem of inquiry" (Fesmire 1995, 570). Moral deliberation, thus, starts from particular problems in order to develop a story. Specifically, particular problems are characterized by conflict with existent conditions. Moral deliberation through imagination works, in part, to develop a coherent story (or "narrative") that adequately "expresses" the conflicts that characterize the particular problem to be solved. And here, it might be best to understand, for moral purposes, the term "coherence" in a particular way.

In James's essay "The Moral Philosopher and the Moral Life," the moral philosopher is anyone who attempts to bring about a coherent moral universe—that is, a world in which we recognize the connection of our desires with those of others in order to fashion a common moral viewpoint. In traditional Western ethical philosophy, moral activity is based on principles of conduct that demand that a person drop her own desires in light of the right and the good, accommodating herself to the prevailing order. On this traditional account, "the other" is never taken seriously as a uniquely desiring individual since all desires come from one universal rational scheme. James, on the other hand, does not develop his account of morality based on a "prevailing order" of things. There is no universal "right" and "good" to which we must accommodate ourselves. "Right" and "good" are the ends of inquiry and moral deliberation, not the beginnings, and as such, will only arise after careful consideration of all persons affected by the current situation and the consequences of our proposed actions. In this light, deliberation by the moral philosopher must attempt to *create* a narrative that includes as many concrete interests as possible. James states succinctly, "*Invent some manner* of realizing your own ideals which will also satisfy the alien demands—that and only that is the path to peace" (James [1897] 1956, 623). In other words, the narrative of the "moral philosopher" should include disparate narratives of her own *and* others. Fesmire, in turn, tells us that is best done by setting ourselves in the place of the other.

[A] "complete" dramatic rehearsal strives to weave the interests and purposes of ourselves and others into an integrated and enduring tapestry. Hence, not only must we forecast consequences for ourselves, but also, as Mead observes, we must (and do) dramatically play the role of others whose lives interlace with our own. We must imaginatively project ourselves into the emerging dramas of *their* lives to discover how their life-stories or "narrative" may be meaningfully continued alongside our own. Immoral conduct is thus not merely a deficiency in one's capacity to follow moral laws or rules. Much more than this, immorality stems from a scarcity of moral imagination and a failure in moral artistry. (Fesmire 1995, 571)

Dewey's dramatic rehearsal in imagination that leads to Fesmire's account of moral artistry through the weaving of Jamesean-style coherent narratives that take the other in one's desires seriously, demands a great deal of work. *Moral activity is not easy.* However, recalling our earlier discussion of intelligent habits and habits of intelligence that lead to pragmatic understanding, we can begin to see that moral artistry is actually the imaginative use of habits of intelligence in everyday social situations. The moral artist never merely attempts to apply abstract rules or principles; that person learns to view problems through habits of intelligence that creatively and dramatically rehearse possible solutions to problematic situations at hand, adjusting desires and the situation in order to develop a story that takes the other seriously. "Deliberation is not a mathematical utilitarian calculation, nor is it a Kantian determinate judgment; it has a dramatic *story to tell*" (Fesmire 1995, 574 [emphasis mine]).

David Burrell and Stanley Hauerwas expand this even further when they say,

> There can be no normative theory of the moral life that is sufficient to capture the rich texture of the many moral notions we inherit. What we actually possess are various and sometimes conflicting stories that provide us with the many skills to use certain moral notions. What we need to develop is the reflective capacity to analyze those stories, so that we better understand how they function. It is not theory-building that develops such a capacity so much as close attention to the ways our distinctive communities tell their stories. (Burrell and Hauerwas 1979, 170)

Burrell and Hauerwas note that morality is not simply about isolated individuals and their desires and stories, but in order to develop moral rationality, we must pay "close attention to the ways our distinctive communities tell their stories." This begins to point to the idea that morality is not about atomic individuals attempting to protect their activities in light of the presence of others (à la John Locke), but is always-already wrapped up in situations of communities. We cannot begin moral deliberation from the standpoint of a fully constituted individual who resides in isolation from all others. James implores us to "invent" some way of taking the other seriously because each of us is not an insular self alone, but a socially situated being who is both creating and created by the communities in which we participate.

SOCIALLY SITUATED SELVES

Since the time of the Enlightenment, Western social/political philosophy has been dominated by a kind of thought known as liberal individualism that gives an account of the self as both prior to, and fundamentally insulated from, society. In the theories of thinkers from Locke to Kant, the self is taken as a well-constituted entity ontologically prior to empirical experiences or social relations. In Locke's philosophy, the idea that moral activity must recognize the autonomy of the individual to be a natural right is central. Kant, on the other hand, explains that the concept of autonomy is a formal necessity for the very possibility of morality. Both moral theories isolate the individual from society, a move (as we shall see in chapter 3) that Alasdair MacIntyre (among others) has both recognized, and, I believe, correctly criticized. Unfortunately, this Enlightenment emphasis on and reification of the insular individual has been passed down to us today in many forms.

It should be easy to see that our own historical American political and philosophical development is deeply rooted in the Enlightenment emphasis on the insular individual. It is nothing new to point out that the ideas and spirit of the Declaration of Independence were greatly influenced by Locke. But note also that Ralph Waldo Emerson's famous essay entitled "Self-Reliance" emphasizes Enlightenment themes of individualism. Henry David Thoreau, Walt Whitman, and Theodore Roosevelt, among others, have all added to the championing of a strong, independent individual. Today, politicians and pundits alike talk of the interference of government in our lives, the fear of socialized medicine, and so on. The American dream itself is characterized by the singular individual who beats the odds, bucks the trend, pulls herself up by the bootstraps, and makes a change or forges on to progress.

Bioethics, too, has taken up the charge of the Enlightenment. As I show in the following two chapters—and specifically in chapter 3—while discussing Beauchamp/Childress's and Engelhardt's principles of autonomy, individualism in the classical sense is at the very foundation of some of the most popular bioethical theories. This principle of autonomy (in all of its many forms) champions the individual over and against, rather than in conjunction with, the beliefs, interests, and desires of others and of society at large. In the biomedical arena, though the principle of autonomy taken negatively does provide an injunction to protect patients from unwanted care, the most it can do in any positive sense is demand that "consent" be given by the patient before any activity is performed; leaving the patient as merely "patient"—that is, as someone upon whom action will be taken.

It is clear that both the great American leaders of the past and the bioethicists of today, in their actions and writings, do show the special and important perspective gained when individualism is applauded over and against other social/political theories; however, we run the risk of falling into a dangerous Enlightenment error constituted by the insularity of the individual, dangerous because we run the risk of leading unintegrated lives, disenfranchised from others, and, paradoxically, from ourselves. Dewey is quite lucid on this topic in his book *Individualism, Old and New*. There, he calls Enlightenment individualism the "older individualism" which is "pre-scientific" and pretechnological; it "anteceded the rise of modern industry and the era of the machine" (LW5, 77). It is, however, incapable of dealing with the changes and movements within society since the early Enlightenment period. As Dewey says, "Such thinking treats individualism as if it were something static, having a uniform content. It ignores the fact that the mental and moral structure of individuals, the pattern of their desires and purposes, change with every great change in social constitution" (LW5, 80).[18] The older individualism opposes the "corporate" and "collective" character of contemporary society while missing the crucial question: "How shall the individual refind himself in an unprecedentedly new social situation, and what qualities will the new individualism exhibit?" (LW5, 81).

To answer Dewey, we shall discuss in chapter 4 the idea that no human comes into the world fully formed; we are socially situated beings always-already in community, being shaped by and shaping our environments. Reason itself is not separate from experience, but arises with habits of experience. As Dewey himself says, "The individual cannot remain intellectually a vacuum [as the older individualism would have it]. If his ideas and beliefs are not the spontaneous function of a communal life in which he shares," activity becomes merely mechanical and artificial (LW5, 81). Individuals are not over-and-against society but are only fully integrated beings when part of a community that helps to shape and mold who they are and further provides outlets for action. Dewey's "new individualism" is "marked by consensus with others . . . [and] sociability . . . [as] cooperation in all regular human associations" (LW5, 84). Enlightenment theories miss this important *inter*play between individual and community, an interplay that arises out of and creates the constitution of the self and the very fabric of experience.

The implications for medical encounters are many. First, contemporary bioethical theories based primarily on Enlightenment conceptions of the self misconstrue the nature of the self, which is evidenced by their reliance on the principle of autonomy. Autonomy in bioethics treats selves as insular, and only provides empowerment for patients through the act of consent, leaving the patient in a rather passive state. However, as a reaction against this notion of the insular individual as it shows itself in contemporary bioethics, chapter 4 will focus on a positive account of the self, not as atomic, but as a product of social interaction. I wish to show, with help from such thinkers as James, Dewey, and Mead, that the self only arises by way of interaction with its environment, both social and natural.[19] The self is not an unchanging entity at the core of each human being, but is a process and function—or as I shall explain, a "narrative"—that develops and changes as individuals learn to adapt to and manipulate the world around them. This narrative self is inextricably tied up in community, situated and saturated with and by others. This leads to the further insight that meaningful, personal, individual ends cannot be pursued in a vacuum; they are tied into a complex series of the ends of others and of the community as a whole. Others are implicated in our actions as conditions for the possibility of those actions. To pursue our ends successfully, then, it would behoove us to develop means that account not only for our own purposes but for those of others as well, engaging them in our activities while necessarily and desirously engaging in theirs.

Of course, as we have already noted above, these pursuits, in order to be moral, take the imaginative moral artistry of creatively intelligent persons. This is an active process of involvement in the current circumstances and future pursuits expressed and required in the situation at hand. Thereby, the engaged participant, and not the passive, consenting patient, becomes our "model" for physicians and patients alike. Together, health care professionals and patients pursue desired ends that, as Pellegrino states, are the right healing actions for particular patients.

Furthermore, in pursuing ends it is important to note that the value of any end attained "is a value of something which in being an end, an outcome, stands in relation to the means of which it is the consequence. Hence, if the object in question is prized *as* an end of 'final' value, it is valued *in this relation*" (LW13, 227 [Dewey's emphasis]). Morally artistic engagements exemplify an important continuum between means and ends, where the goals we pursue and the activities performed to pursue them are not taken in isolation from one another. Our moral deliberations shape the outcomes we achieve and vice versa. Ethical medical encounters that engage the patient in her own healing process, making her a participant in the health care community, typify this means–end continuum, for (as I will argue in chapter 5) if health is nothing else, it is surely the active participation of the individual within the communities of which that person is a part.

COMMUNITY AS HEALING

By developing positive accounts of both intelligent moral artistry and communally situated selves, we will then have new tools with which to approach ethical issues in physician–patient relationships. These tools help break down the model of the insular self. Beginning in chapter 4 with a discussion of meaningful living and participation in one's own life story, I show in chapter 5 that meaningful living, though it takes on many forms, is important from birth to death, and that significance in life is only possible by engaging others, by participating in community.

These insights illustrate that the life of an individual is a communal process, and that the lives of patients must be also. They demand that in medical encounters, physicians engage their patients in morally imaginative ways. We will find that the moral minimum of "informed consent" championed by Beauchamp/Childress and Engelhardt is simply not enough, morally or practically, for positive, progressive human interaction and participation. What is required is recognition that we are socially situated beings who define health as what Richard Zaner calls the "taken-for-granted" quality of experience. Healthy living is the common *participation* in, with, and by community. It is the significant, meaningful *engagement* in one's pursuits within a social context. Therefore, living significantly in community should be both the end and means of most medical encounters. As chapter 5 will argue, to put it oversimply, a meaningful life integrates both individual and social aspects of life, where socially situated individuals actively participate in the life stories of themselves and their communities. And, *since living in community with others*—that is, living healthily—*is the end-in-view for medical encounters, it too must be implicated in the means to that end.* This dismisses "autonomy," in any Enlightenment sense of "atomic selves," as our basic moral model in medical encounters (in any encounter, really) and instead takes "community" as healing.

NOTES

1. Many twentieth-century educators of medicine and medical history clearly illustrate this trend. For example, Abraham Flexner, in his book based on a 1910 report concerning the status and future of medical education in North America, states that medicine is a blend of superstition, empiricism, and science. We must endeavor to make it truly scientific to the exclusion of superstition and empiricism. Science is the effort to "purify, extend, and organize knowledge . . . undoubtedly the more accurately — or mathematically — [we do it] . . . the better" (Flexner 1925, 3). This focus on pure science leads later authors like Henry Sigerist to state that preparation for medical school should be based in physics, chemistry, biology, bacteriology, mathematics, and psychology. "Medicine as research is its final and ultimate stage" (Sigerist 1951, 310). And more contemporary leaders of medicine continue this legacy. As noted by Professor Charles Odegaard while commenting on the 1984 presidential address of Dr. John D. Cooper to the American Association of Medical Colleges, "One cannot escape the conclusion that in [Dr. Cooper's] Report the Flexnerian form of medical education with its exclusive concentration on disease as simply a malfunction of the organs and tissues of the body interpreted in light of findings based on the biological, chemical, and physical sciences was accepted without the need for comment" (White 1988, 100).

2. Of course, it is not as simple as this. For one, this begs the question of whether patients were ever seen by physicians (or even themselves) as active participants in their own health care. The "doctor knows best" style of paternalism was clearly a factor long before World War II. At the same time, however, for many Americans, their doctors were well known to them, made house calls, were available around the clock. Today, most physicians are only seen in clinics, and the rise of medical centers and HMOs has produced a great distancing between physicians and patients on a personal level. Couple this with the "disease" paradigm still holding sway in much of medicine today, and the relationship between physician and patient is tenuous and lopsided.

3. See Fletcher 1954 and Ramsey 1970.

4. In particular, Dr. Henry Beecher at Harvard; see Beecher 1966. Further, for a discussion of the history of bioethics as well as Beecher's, Fletcher's, and Ramsey's places in it, see Rothman 1991.

5. It is interesting to note that even an ethicist like Gregory Pence begins his account with a two-and-one-half page description of Barnard while offering less than a page on Washkansky, and one-half page on the donor, Denise Darvall.

Also, an explosion of transplants occurred in the year following Barnard's transplant: 105 heart transplants and 55 liver transplants. Fewer than 6 percent lived longer than 6 months after their operations.

6. For a brief description of this case, see Munson 2000 (190–92). For a discussion of the historical impact of this case, see Rothman 1991 (222–46). For a discussion of some of the ethical issues in this case, see (among others) Pence 2000 (29–38). For a legal perspective, see Annas 1988 (261–66).

7. I realize that it may not be the case that the theories of Beauchamp/Childress and Engelhardt had any direct influence on the development of these formal procedures. Further, it is obvious that the bioethicists used an ethical vocabulary already somewhat familiar to the health care professional. This does not diminish the fact, however, that since 1979, the discipline of bioethics has been governed by the agenda set by these thinkers, and as bioethics has become a more visible part of the clinic, physicians' use of the vocabulary of autonomy and beneficence has not been questioned so much as it has been validated.

8. This has been changing slowly in the last half decade. Several contemporary bioethicists do have firm roots in the soil of classical American thought—for example, Mary Briody Mahowald, Jonathan Moreno, John Lachs, John J. McDermott, Glenn McGee, Griffin Trotter, and a few others. And even though in recent years, professional meetings have provided forums for so-called "pragmatic bioethics," unfortunately, pragmatism-based writings are still, for the most part (Mahowald's writings, e.g., are notable exceptions), left out of the mainstream collections in medical ethics. Interestingly, in a published lecture on the history of bioethics in the last thirty years, noted bioethicist Albert Jonsen concluded his remarks with what he calls his "philosophical fantasy": "Many of us have wondered how the desiccated moral philosophy of the 1960s turned into the vigorous ethics of bioethics. . . . My fantasy is that the ghost of our two great American philosophers, William James and John Dewey, silently presided over the transformation. . . . It is my impression that philosophers who have become bioethicists have followed, *unknowingly*, the lead of these preeminent American philosophers" (Jonsen 1997, 19 [emphasis mine]). Jonsen himself, even in his coauthored book *The Abuse of Casuistry*, rarely mentioned either James or Dewey in his own writings, but in this speech before the Society for Health and Human Values (1996), he makes the startling pronouncement that they have been there in the background all the time, and not only in his work but in most all of American bioethics. However, what is apparent even in these comments is that this influence by James and Dewey is still "unknown" and underappreciated.

9. A previous version (now much revised) of the following section was used in Hester 1999.

10. Throughout this book I will use terms like "medical practitioners," "health care professionals," and "physicians" interchangeably and do so to highlight that many of the issues discussed herein apply in varying degrees to M.D.'s, D.O.'s, R.N.'s, P.T.'s, and others, alike. Certainly (as I argue below), particular moral responsibilities fall squarely on the shoulders of physicians because of their asymmetrically powerful positions in health care delivery, but the community of health care includes all medical personnel, administrators, and, of course, patients themselves. Thus, many of the roadblocks to building this community must be addressed to and by all those who should be working to develop the community.

11. We possibly could stretch this point beyond the world of human making and doing, but I need not be so bold for the subject matter at hand.

12. See particularly chapter 4 in James [1890] 1950, and part 1, among others, in MW14.

13. See especially chapter 25.

14. This comes from a conversation I had with a Columbia/HCA director who recounted the events of a business retreat at which Rick Scott (former CEO of

Columbia/HCA) made a statement to the effect that in the three areas of business practices—
service, innovation, and operational efficiency—Columbia was primarily to focus its efforts
on operational efficiency. The director, by the way, agreed with Mr. Scott on this point.

15. Sociologists Raymond DeVries and Peter Conrad have pointed out that bioethicists
themselves have paid far too little attention to the institutional environments in which
medical practice becomes habituated and supported. See DeVries and Conrad 1998 (in
particular 235–37). I fear that this book, too, does not go very far in this regard and shall
need supplementary support with further work on what might be called "sociological
bioethics of medical institutions" in future writings.

16. A panel discussion of these very diagnostic computer applications occurred in 1978,
and updated papers based on that conference were published seven years later in the book
Logic of Discovery and Diagnosis in Medicine (Schaffner 1985).

17. This is not to imply that a naive and unreflective approach has been taken to the development of these computer applications. Quite the contrary, great care has been taken
and thoughtful debate has been considered in order to account for concerns of logicians,
physicians, philosophers, and patients. However, important and regrettable reductionism
by the computer (at this stage of technology) is inevitable.

18. Dewey makes this critique elsewhere as well (cf. LW11, 30).

19. Pragmatists are certainly not the only thinkers who have argued for a conception of
the self as socially situated, though they may have been doing so for a longer period of
time than others. Many feminist theorists, existential psychologists, and sociologists of
race and sexuality (among others) have all made similar points, particularly in the last half
century.

Chapter 2

Principles and Pragmatism: Negative Considerations for Positive Beginnings

INTRODUCTION

Given the positive force behind this book—that is, the attempt to bring classical American philosophy to bear on bioethics and professional–patient encounters—a thorough exploration of contemporary bioethics is impractical and unnecessary. I do not intend, therefore, to discuss every movement in contemporary bioethics. "Principlism," "casuistry," "virtue ethics," and so on all have their proponents and opponents. However, in order to establish a context for my position concerning ethical practices within physician–patient relationships, it is useful to look at what is still quite possibly the most influential approach to contemporary bioethics: the use of basic bioethical principles, and particularly in the next chapter, the principle of autonomy (or "respect for autonomy" or even "permission").[1]

Though so-called principlism[2] "has been assaulted, criticized, and amended by a host of critics . . . it [has been] . . . adopted as the standard approach to bioethical issues, its seminal contribution is widely acknowledged, and its vocabulary and basic principles remain at the center of bioethical debate" (Wolpe 1998, 41). And, more importantly, it has become the basis of conversations with and among health care professionals concerning the ethical issues they face in their clinical practices.

There is, however, a danger in taking on ethical issues beginning at the level of principles. I will show that any appeal to principles is ultimately vacuous or, at the very least, skeletal. As this chapter evolves, we will move from an explanation of the use of principles in bioethics to a critique of this approach. In this light, this and the following chapters' purposes are primarily negative; however, we cannot lose sight of the fact that their negative conclusions concerning principlism are for the further purpose of establishing in chapter 4 a positive ethical alternative to appeals to the principle of autonomy for health care professionals and patients—namely, a pragmatic method of intelligent moral artistry performed by and for socially situated selves.

21

BEAUCHAMP AND CHILDRESS: PRINCIPLES AND SPECIFICATIONS

In 1979, Tom Beauchamp and James Childress published the first edition of their landmark work in contemporary bioethics, *Principles of Biomedical Ethics*. By the publication of the fourth edition of *Principles* in 1994, the work had become "one of the most important basic texts for medical ethics."[3] Though some changes have occurred between the first and fourth editions (we will note a few later), in each incarnation, the authors argue for an approach to biomedical ethics based on the use of four basic principles: autonomy (in the fourth edition this becomes "respect for autonomy"), nonmaleficence, beneficence, and justice.[4] The principle of autonomy obligates physicians to allow patients to give consent before any procedures are performed. As a restatement of the Hippocratic dictum "do no harm," the principle of nonmaleficence urges that physicians should avoid harmful treatment of their patients. The principle of beneficence is the reverse (or "positive") side of nonmaleficence and states that physicians should attempt to "do good" or benefit their patients—that is, look out for a patient's "best interests." Lastly, the principle of justice expresses that physicians are bound to give each patient her due or "dessert." According to Beauchamp and Childress, "for biomedical ethics, which has concentrated on guidelines for action, principles and rules are both indispensable and central to the enterprise" (PBE 1994, 40). Ethically problematic situations in medicine are best approached by way of an application of one or more of these principles in order to clarify and, ultimately, solve the problems arising therein.[5]

Certainly, it would seem at first glance that such general principles are in line with commonsense notions—that is, if we *all* do indeed share the same common sense as Beauchamp and Childress. For example, patients should be allowed, whenever possible and wherever it is determined to be just, to make their own choices, avoid being harmed, and ultimately be benefited by medical treatment. But with these all-too-brief descriptions, it is easy to envision situations for which these principles might be too vague to help or may, in fact, conflict with each other. Take, for example, the case of an elderly patient with advanced Alzheimer's; recognition of others, of time and place, of self becomes difficult if not impossible. How can we appropriately apply the principle of autonomy when the patient's decision-making capacity is, at best, suspect or compromised? Or in the case of organ transplantation where more than 74,000 people are waiting for hard organ transplants (for example, more than 48,000 are waiting for kidneys, alone), who "deserves" any specific donated organ, and on what factors can we ethically base our decision?[6] Consider situations of physician-assisted suicide where conflicts between beneficence and nonmaleficence abound, and the very definitions of "harm" and "benefit" are in question: How can physicians both follow their Hippocratic obligations and yet turn a deaf ear to the pleadings of terminally ill and degenerating individuals?

In order to address just these types of problems, the authors do not leave the definitions and explanations of these principles to simplified, brief statements. Each principle receives a chapter devoted to its elaboration in order to clarify its use. (However, we shall see later, as exemplified by the case for the "principle of autonomy," these discussions do little to fill in the details.)[7] While I am primarily concerned here with how Beauchamp and Childress use their principles, before I can discuss that, I need briefly to explore the theoretical origins of these principles.

The Theory

Beginning with a focus on human practices and activities, Beauchamp and Childress explain that the creation of ethical principles arises out of our social norms or "communal consensus" concerning conventions of conduct. This communal consensus is embodied in us as, what philosopher John Rawls calls, "considered judgments" (cf. Rawls 1971), which are "the moral convictions in which we have the highest confidence and believe to have the lowest level of bias" (PBE 1994, 20), and these considered judgments "are acceptable initially without argumentative support" (PBE 1994, 24). Considered judgments seem, then, to be shared, communal beliefs that are acceptable to all without need for immediate justification (implying that they may need justification at some later time depending on the deliberation at hand). They form the basis for reflection when new problems arise. Not unlike pragmatist convictions, Beauchamp and Childress recognize that de facto we begin in experience with a stockpile of habits of judgment and action. The question is, then, how are new judgments made when novel situations confront us? It is the answer to this question that begins to divide Beauchamp and Childress from a pragmatist position.

Using Rawls's notion of "reflective equilibrium" (an adjustment of considered judgments to ethical principles, and on Rawlsian terms, at least, vice versa) in order to develop a "coherentism," Beauchamp and Childress explain, "The goal of reflective equilibrium is to match, prune, and adjust considered judgments so that they coincide and are rendered coherent with the premises of theory. That is, we start with paradigm judgments of moral rightness and wrongness, and then construct a more general theory that is consistent with these paradigm judgments" (PBE 1994, 21).[8] Ethical principles, thus, are put forth, which give a rational reconstruction of our considered judgments. In turn, the considered judgments may, through a reflection on the implications of the principles, be changed in order to comply more closely with the principles themselves. For Beauchamp and Childress, the use of reflective equilibrium on our communal consensus helps determine a theory of "common morality" that "takes its basic premises directly from the morality shared in common by the members of a society—that is, unphilosophical common sense and tradition" (PBE 1994, 100). Beauchamp and Childress believe their principles to be rooted in common sense, and develop a theory of "common morality" out of this belief while accepting that these principles clearly arise from a shared morality.

Again, there is much here with which a pragmatist like myself can agree. Reflection must take place on both sides of the equation. There seems to be both a movement from experience to theory and a movement back to experience with adjustments at both ends. It is, however, importantly and dangerously misleading to speak in this way given that the "two movements" are neither independent of each other nor neatly "linear" or exclusive in their developments. Beauchamp and Childress's language betrays them when they speak of the activities of "reflective equilibrium" that start not at the level of particular experiences and judgments but at the level of "paradigm" judgments (judgments already abstracted from particular experiences). From there, considered judgments are items "matched and pruned" in order to "render [them] coherent with the premises of theory" and *not* vice versa. They speak most pointedly to the "second movement" down from ethical theory, adjusting considered judgments to principles, but not principles to judgments.

As we have begun to see, then, though it has points of contact with the pragmatists, Beauchamp and Childress's explanation of the origin and status of principles quickly loses this connection. They say that "[t]he principles [are] *embedded* in these shared moral beliefs" (PBE 1994, 100 [emphasis mine]), and a page later, they state that their "strategy allows [them] to rely on *the authority of the indispensable principles* in the common morality" (PBE 1994, 101 [emphasis mine]). These statements alone imply an a priori nature that is discoverable in our judgments as well as a fundamental necessity of the principles to any moral enterprise. That is, the principles are described as already implied by our shared beliefs and *cannot* be discarded. Once they are proposed as *the* basic bioethical principles, reflective adjustment of them is never considered a rational possibility. Beauchamp and Childress seem to take for granted that they have discovered "authoritative" and "indispensable" tools for any medically based ethical inquiry; they make the move from considered judgments up to principles and then throw away the ladder, claiming that they have found the starting point for investigation clearly implied by our experienced judgments in the first place.

Further, in the introductory chapter of the first edition, we learn that generally speaking, the use of principles is a deductive process. As such, in our ethical practice, we must justify our actions by beginning at a high level of abstraction from particular cases and work our way down through various rules and specifications derived from the principles (which are themselves based on ethical theory) in order to apply any principle to a particular context. "[J]udgments about what ought to be done in particular situations are justified by moral rules, which in turn are grounded in principles and ultimately in ethical theories" (PBE 1979, 5). That is, we derive the justification for our particular actions from the rules and principles upon which they are based. Since it has been determined by Beauchamp and Childress that the rules and principles of bioethics enframe all good medical practice, then our actions must be good so long as they follow directly from the principles.

It should be noted, however, that by the fourth edition, the authors believe that this deductivist approach only "functions smoothly whenever a judgment can be brought directly under a rule or principle without intervening complexities such as appeals to several principles" (PBE 1994, 16). Instead of continuing to commit to the deductive method, they offer their Rawlsian-style coherence theory as an alternative to deductivism. For that matter, Beauchamp and Childress further claim that they steer clear of any account that moves only from particular experience up to high-level principles and theory—that is, inductivism. In order to navigate this difficult terrain, their approach contains three "safeguards" that they assert are necessary to any "coherence" model of norms: (1) the resemblance condition—any moral account must "resemble" its starting principles and "considered judgments," (2) universalizability—any action deemed morally right in a given circumstance is morally right in any other given circumstance provided there is no morally relevant difference between the circumstances, and (3) endurance and adaptivity—any coherent set of moral norms must be long term and able to deal with novel situations.

Though this is obviously not a straightforward deductivist approach, the first two safeguards (resemblance and universalizability) do have both deductivist and Kantian overtones that bring into question the practical difference between the Beauchamp and Childress coherence theory and deductivism. Far too much hangs on what is meant by either "resemblance" or what constitutes a "morally relevant difference." They begin as inductivists from the point of view of "theory construction," but once constructed, and protestations to the contrary, their justifications for moral activity are based solely on deduction from the four "indispensable" principles.

Their coherence theory and deductivism are brought even more closely in line when these safeguards lead Beauchamp and Childress to introduce the method of "specification" that is established to help derive appropriate actions from general principles. They say, "Obviously, no body of abstract principles and rules can dictate policy [or action], because it cannot contain enough specific information or provide direct and discerning guidance" (PBE 1994, 10; cf. PBE 1979, 12). Since principles themselves are not capable of guiding specific action, the authors introduce the practice of "specification" where general principles are made useful by "specify[ing] the content in a way that surpasses ethereal abstractness, while also indicating the cases that properly fall under the principles" (PBE 1994, 28).[9] These "specifications" of principles (1) are based on considered judgments, (2) must "resemble" the principles they specify, and (3) must fit coherently with other specifications. One example given is that in order for physicians to follow rules against "deception," they must recognize that following these rules might conflict with other legal and moral rules. Using the case of falsifying insurance forms in order to pay for diagnostic and therapeutic means, Beauchamp and Childress attempt to show that physicians "specify" rules against deception by such means as writing that a mammography exam is intended to "rule out cancer" as opposed to being merely "routine" in order to get insurance to cover the costs. Through these acts, physicians show that they operate under a "specific" definition of the rule against deception and their actions are rendered "coherent" with other moral rules—for example, "Doctors should put their patients' interests first" (PBE 1994, 29–30).[10]

Beyond this, however, Beauchamp and Childress explain little else about the use of specifications. We do not know which judgments to accept without question; we are not given a way to measure "resemblance" or even told what "resemblance" might mean here, and we are not told how to recognize adequate coherence. Even with these questions unanswered and continuing to show their deductivist stripes, they feel,

> The upshot of our analysis of coherence and specification is the following: One goal of moral theory, and central to its account of justification, is *to move from general levels of theory to particular rules, judgments, and policies that are in close proximity* to everyday decisions in the moral life. (PBE 1994, 31 [emphasis mine])

At this point, at least two important and related problems arise: (1) there is an admitted danger in beginning from high-level abstraction since at such a level no context exists, yet every problem that we confront always-already arises as a *particular* problem happening to *particular* people in some *unique context*, and (2) since Beauchamp and Childress already recognize the inability of principles to aid directly in dictating specific action, why do they insist on justifying all activity from the level of abstract principles and not through reflection on specific problems?[11] Clearly, they believe that their approach accounts for common sense. However, with no attempt to question radically the authority of their principles (even after fifteen years and four editions) and with no appeal to actual lived experience once the principles have been established, for all intents and purposes particular contexts play little or no role in their notion of ethical medical practice.

A Response to a "Logical" Error

The pragmatist John Dewey is alert to just these kinds of problems when he says,

> Beginning with definitions, rules, general principles, classifications, and the like is a common form of the . . . error [of isolation of deduction at the beginning of inquiry]. . . . [T]he mistake is, logically, due to the attempt to introduce deductive considerations without first making acquaintance with the particular facts that create a need for the generalizing rational devices. (MW6, 98–99)

Inquiry in general, and ethical inquiry in particular, arises out of a given problematic situation. There are specific features, details, and occurrences that make up the subject matter of any inquiry. By isolating the "two movements" of inquiry from each other as Beauchamp and Childress do, they have no recourse but to approach any new problematic situation from a purely deductivist standpoint. Since inquiry begins within *some* content-filled problematic situation making itself felt and present to us, Beauchamp and Childress are, then, committing the "logical" error Dewey warns of by attempting to begin first with principles that are abstract and *without* content. We cannot move from general principles if we are not first acquainted with the specific features of the problem at hand, and any appropriate ethical principle must arise out of the context if it is to have any meaning to the given situation. *Principles must be developed from the features and specifics of the problematic situation that we are attempting to make satisfactory.*

Beauchamp and Childress fall prey to this logical error the moment they profess to develop principles and rules that they admit "may appear to be distant from both history and contemporary problems in the biological sciences, medicine, nursing, and other modes of health care" (PBE 1994, 3). Ethical discussions of the many different practices of health care professionals must not be "distant from" those practices, but rooted in them. Contrary to their own take on the matter, Beauchamp and Childress separate and isolate from each other the movements from practice to theory and back. They develop distant principles that they *apply* to medical contexts in order to determine appropriate moral actions. Ethical justification is made only by way of the deductivist slide from theory down to practice. And yet they frequently admit the inadequacy of their discussion without some particular context in which to operate.[12] This, of course, raises the second problem, for if they recognize that principles are useless without further specifications, why begin with principles at all? What ethical work do principles do for specific cases? As they say, "*In difficult cases*, direct application [of principles] rarely works. . . . Specification, then is an attractive strategy for the hard cases as long as the specification can be justified" (PBE 1994, 29 [emphasis mine]).

An immediate concern arises at this point: What kind of cases are we worried about in (bio)ethics if not so-called "difficult cases"? Every problem is initially, at least, experienced as difficult or else we would not perceive it to be a problem. If we already saw the case as easy, no question concerning how to approach it would arise. Each medical encounter takes place with particular people in a particular place and time. Individuals come together in order to solve a unique medical problem. Of course, from the perspective of disease classification, we might question what is "unique" about some patient contracting breast cancer or Parkinson's disease since it is the case that many people throughout the ages have also contracted such medical conditions. However, from the perspective of the patient and her experienced illness, there should be no question concerning the uniqueness of any particular case of, for example, HIV for a particular person (whether it be Magic Johnson or some young mother-to-be) since that case affects specific individuals with unique relationships, status, gender issues, cultural ties, expressed desires, and obligations. All of our inquiries (medical, ethical, etc.) in situations related to health care must look for, as stated by Edmund Pellegrino in the previous chapter, "a decision 'good' for *this* patient" (Pellegrino 1979, 173 [emphasis mine]). Ethical and clinical decisions begin with particular individuals "as . . . knowing and valuing beings" (Pellegrino 1979, 174). Certainly, we are looking for patterns, "signs," symptoms, and so forth; they stand as questions to be asked and conditions to be examined. But these arise *because of*, and must be taken up into the concrete situation. Any use of principles or classifications, then, can only happen given a specific problem and context or "[g]iven the signs and symptoms presented by *this* patient" (Pellegrino 1979, 174 [emphasis mine]). From an ethical and clinical standpoint, one consequence that follows from a "principlist" theory is that uniqueness between situations and individuals is prima facie ignored, difference is washed out, only later to find that particular specifications need to be made in order to use effectively the general principles. What minimal content the principle might contain—for example, "let someone choose for herself" or "do no harm"—gets supplanted by some further clarification based on the specific issues of a particular case. Clearly, this then begs the question of the effective need for these four basic bioethical principles at all.

Fundamentally, then, the question at hand is the status and function of principles of ethics in general and bioethics in particular. It is a matter of cultural history that appeal to and use of principles exists in ethical inquiry. Bioethics has simply taken up the use of ethical principles, which is not in itself troubling. However, Beauchamp and Childress place a priority on principles that limits ethical inquiry and disables communication. While the world to which they apply and the human beings whom they help guide continue to evolve (both biologically and culturally), the principles seemingly remain unchanged. They reside outside the specific operations and situations of people and things. *If difficulties arise in given empirical situations, however, why start outside the situations at the level of abstract principles only to come back to the particulars of the situations in order to make the principles useful?*

The problem is clear; principles lose touch with individuals and their specific values and interests. They do not account for differences among individuals and situations. One way to solve this problem is to reconstruct our conception of principles and reevaluate their use and status, their origin and function. However, although I will briefly take this approach at the end of this chapter, I will opt primarily to move away from the language and use of principles altogether and instead attempt to reconstruct our notions of individual and of community later in chapters 4 and 5.

The above should make clear my objections to Beauchamp and Childress's appeal to and use of four general principles of biomedical ethics. However, they are not the only major players in bioethics who rely on an appeal to a set of principles, and where their approach failed, maybe others have succeeded. For example, whereas the so-called principlism of Beauchamp and Childress focuses on four major principles, H. Tristram Engelhardt uses only two: autonomy and beneficence. Also, whereas the former authors attempt to wade between empiricism and rationalism, utilitarianism and deontology, the latter develops an overtly Kantian, formalist approach. It is to this account of principles, then, that I turn next.

ENGELHARDT: PRINCIPLES FOR A SECULAR PLURALIST SOCIETY

Seven years after the publication of Beauchamp and Childress's famous work, another important text in bioethics was published. The first edition of *The Foundations of Bioethics* (1986) by Engelhardt came out to a very receptive audience. (Ten years later, a second edition of this highly influential "standard" of bioethics literature was also published.) In his work, Engelhardt argues that since the Reformation, the possibility of a common moral viewpoint has been lost. Martin Luther's ninety-five theses, the Pax Westphalica that ended the Thirty Years' War, and the Copernican revolution all moved to "leave us devoid of a sense of absolute or final perspective: man was to cease to be the center of the cosmos, and the established Christian view of the cosmos was to be overturned" (FB 1986, 3).

According to Engelhardt, contemporary society inherits this radical metaphysical and moral transformation. We are children of the Enlightenment who live in what Engelhardt terms a secular pluralist society—"secular" in that no religious institution or doctrine has final authority within a democracy, and "pluralist" in that democratic societies encompass diverse (even competing) moral viewpoints. This has led to what Engelhardt calls a "secular ethic" where no single viewpoint is put forth, but where any viewpoint "available to rational individuals" is allowed. "The history of bioethics [itself] over the last two decades has been the story of a secular ethic. . . . Bioethics is an element of secular culture and the great-grandchild of the Enlightenment" (FB 1986, 5).

While noting the problems of Enlightenment philosophy as pointed out by contemporary thinkers like Alasdair MacIntyre and claiming to oppose the secular pluralist ethic, Engelhardt "endeavor[s] to find grounds for establishing by reason a particular view of the good life and securing by general rational arguments the authority for its establishment" (FB 1986, viii). Without a singular moral authority available in a secular pluralism, we have no ultimately defensible position from which to make particular moral value judgments concerning any specific activity. In order to solve this problem, Engelhardt adopts a Kantian/Rawlsian philosophical position: "[Philosophy] is an endeavor to look at reasons and to determine what reasons should be credited by impartial, unprejudiced, nonculturally biased reasoners, whose only interests are in the consistency and force of rational argument" (FB 1986, 10). Though Engelhardt does state that, ultimately, this endeavor "cannot ground a concrete ethic" (FB 1986, 10) and has much to say in the second edition concerning a critique of the Rawlsian position (see FB 1996, 50-64), it is precisely this Kantian/Rawlsian position that leads him to advocate two principles of bioethics: (1) the principle of autonomy (in the second edition, this is known as the "principle of permission," though substantially nothing changes), and (2) the principle of beneficence.[13]

The Theory (?)

Whereas for Beauchamp and Childress, the principles of biomedical ethics are based on an ethical theory of "common morality" that attempts to adjudicate between Immanuel Kant's deontology and John Stuart Mill's utilitarianism, Engelhardt claims (dubiously) no such theoretical support. As a matter of fact, Engelhardt carefully attempts not to embrace overtly any particular moral viewpoint or theory (though he has a clearly Kantian ethic). Rather, his position is that his two principles are solely based on the *demands* of morality within a secular pluralist society. A secular pluralist society, according to Engelhardt, is made up of both moral friends and moral strangers. Moral friends are found in communities where common norms and beliefs are shared among its members "so that they can resolve moral controversies by sound argument or appeal to a jointly recognized moral authority"—for example, the Catholic community of religious believers (FB 1996, 7). "Moral strangers [on the other hand], are persons who do not share sufficient moral premises . . . to resolve moral controversies by sound rational argument" (FB 1996, 7). Since moral friends agree about particular moral issues, a secular ethic must attempt to adjudicate a position where moral strangers can come together in a peaceful moral community, where moral authority can be developed between differing moral viewpoints. In particular, the principle of autonomy/permission is taken by Engelhardt to be "the necessary condition for the possibility of resolving moral disputes between moral strangers with moral authority and for sustaining a minimum secular ethical language of praise and blame. It is in this sense formal. It provides the empty process for generating moral authority in a secular pluralist society through mutual agreement" (FB 1996, 109).[14]

As for the second principle, beneficence:

> Unlike the principle of permission [autonomy], which justifies the process for generating content, the principle of beneficence identifies the content of the practice of morality. The principle of permission shows that patients may not be used as means merely; the principle of beneficence supports the concrete moral goals to which medicine ought to be directed. (FB 1996, 108)

The principle of beneficence states that we must look to benefit others and ourselves in our actions, though, as Engelhardt points out, in a secular pluralist society, no one "good" can be specified ahead of time. Thus, the principle of beneficence becomes a "somewhat vacuous" deontological requirement of moral action (FB 1996, 115). But why this requirement of beneficence at all? Well, Engelhardt believes that "a concrete understanding of the good life presupposes an ordering, vision, or understanding of goods and harms. . . . As a consequence, morality in a secular pluralist society is the practice of doing good within the bounds of moral authority across communities with disparate moral visions" (FB 1996, 115).

To simplify, it is in community that content for "the good" is given. A moral community is founded on two "necessary conditions . . . (1) an interest in pursuing the good and avoiding harm within (2) the constraints of moral authority, that is permission [autonomy]" (FB 1996, 115). In other words, if we are to commit ourselves to particular moral activities, we must already embrace both the principle of beneficence and the principle of permission/autonomy. "The principle of permission marks the very boundary of all moral communities. To violate it is to be an enemy of moral communities generally. . . . [However,] it is only in affirming the principle of beneficence that one commits oneself to the enterprise of fashioning a moral community and to giving content to beneficence" (FB 1996, 115).

For Engelhardt, then, these two principles work together to help form a moral community in which moral activity—that is, peaceable interaction and tolerance—can occur, bridging the gap between different moral viewpoints. Both principles are deontological and contractual in nature and practice, as is made obvious by Engelhardt's construction of tables of systematic definitions for each principle. In his definitional outline, Engelhardt gives both principles in the form of maxims: (1) "Do not do to others that which they would not have done unto them, and do for them that which one has contracted to do" (autonomy/permission); (2) "Do to others their good [*sic*]" (beneficence) (FB 1986, 85–87; FB 1996, 122–24). As maxims, the principles express formal imperatives for moral conduct.

A Response to Empty Formalism

Again, there are points of agreement between Engelhardt and myself that I do not wish to overlook casually. Engelhardt's recognition of de facto pluralism is well documented and quite laudable. The pragmatist William James would himself agree readily with this insight. And no doubt, it is this de facto pluralism that contributes to the difficulty in developing moral viewpoints from which to adjudicate problematic situations. Further, Engelhardt clearly identifies that morality demands community and that moral goods can only be found in communities. However, a pragmatist quickly parts company with Engelhardt's solution to the problems of morality raised by pluralism and with his rather weak sense of community, not to mention the problems that arise from the formal nature of his principles.

First, Engelhardt's pluralism does not seem genuine, given that his brand of pluralism is reducible to two types of relationships: "moral friends" and "moral strangers." As such, the basic pressing problem for pluralism is how to deal with confrontations between moral strangers. But surely, there is a much richer continuum of "moral" relationships that exists between these two extremes. Engelhardt's take on the matter implies that communities are insular and static. As one of Engelhardt's commentators notes, "There are many moral communities [that is, collections of moral friends] in our society [according to Engelhardt], but there is very little overlap of moral views between them. For the most part these communities are morally isolated from each other" (Strong 1997, 41). Engelhardt's take is, clearly, too black-and-white. Though it seems that he believes that we can be members of multiple communities, this very fact creates at least the possibility for situations that place moral "acquaintances" (neither friends nor strangers) into common moral deliberation.[15] Furthermore, communities are not static entities but are constructed by individuals just as individuals are constructed by them. Again, the changing aspects of communities greatly enhance the chance that a wide variety of "moral" relationships come into play.

Second, Engelhardt's conception of community is rather weak in that he ultimately believes that communities are developed out of contractual relationships with others. According to Engelhardt, moral communities are founded upon "agreement" of the participants who mutually recognize the right of each member to consent to participate in the community. Moral communities exist only if the necessary condition for their possibility, the principle of autonomy (permission), is accepted by all members. As I shall argue in chapter 4, *communities are both more fundamental and more complex* than this. Engelhardt, I shall argue, essentially reverses the equation. It is more true to say that communities are the necessary conditions for autonomy than the other way around, and since communities are actual, organic, empirical realities, morality begins in experience, not outside it. And here I am led to my last point.

Engelhardt takes the Kantian position that the only place to ground morality is prior to experience rather than within it. In this way, Engelhardt attempts to "step behind" experience while a pragmatist like myself does not believe this is possible. Further, by transcending the empirical conditions of society through his use of principles, Engelhardt moves away from and not into morally problematic conditions and, therefore, resolutions. The purely formal nature of his principles, like Kant's before him, begs the question: How is it possible to transcend experience and moral situations long enough to recognize the necessary conditions for them? Though thought experiments are important, they ultimately must reach ground in experience, not beyond it.

According to this explanation, then, Engelhardt's formalism fares little better than the principlism of Beauchamp and Childress. However, before I leave the investigation of these different authors altogether, I wish to revisit and elaborate upon my general critique of the use of principles by both Beauchamp/Childress and Engelhardt.

REVISITING A CRITIQUE OF THE USE OF PRINCIPLES

As we have already begun to see, my position concerning moral rationality differs greatly from both the principlism of Beauchamp and Childress and the formalism of Engelhardt. On my pragmatic account, moral deliberation is an imaginative process of investigation and creation that begins with problematic situations that call for satisfactory resolutions. Difficulties mobilize within us intelligent habits and habits of intelligence in order to develop solutions that both arise out of the specific features of the situation and attempt to bring our habits to bear on them. Though we might say that moral deliberation emphasizes aspects of the situation that primarily concern social interactions and the consequential impact of our actions on others, aside from a difference in emphasis, it does not differ from any other intelligent activity (or activity of intelligence).

Take, for example, a case not heavily laden with medical or moral issues. One day several years ago while I was living in Seattle and working at Kinko's Copies in the University district, I was leaving a small card and gift shop across the street from my place of business. As it was the end of my lunch break, I began to walk back to my store. Giving little thought to the task, since I had walked the streets around my store every day for the past three months, I was abruptly interrupted, physically stopped by some impediment. For a moment, I was taken out of my thoughts as I stood there bewildered. Quickly, however, my eyes focused on what I then realized was a parking meter, one of many that lined the street. After assessing that I had walked into the parking meter and realizing that I needed to step around it in order to cross the street, I was able to make my way to the store, a bit embarrassed at my clumsiness.

As stated in the previous chapter, our considered ethical activity, like that of skirting a parking meter, is the result of reflective thought and habit. It is, in the broadest sense of the terms, both logical and cultural. When we are confronted with a dilemma, we inquire into the situation, we call forth our standing reserve of habits, we mobilize our faculties. This process is evolutionary and reconstructive. We take the subject matter at hand (the physical impediment, an afternoon in the University district, the habit of walking the same street every day, and so on) and our existing conceptions and operative principles (parking meter, inability to walk through solid physical objects) and adjust these factors in order to fashion an appropriate solution (walk around the damn thing). The problem confronted is novel, if only in our immediate confrontation with it. We then attempt to fit this novel situation into our already existing conceptions. These conceptions are previously developed categories and beliefs that function to give meaning to the particular experiences of our daily lives. The impediment in my story gets recognized (re-*cognized* and classified) as "parking meter," which in turn fits with my now-reflected-upon previous experiences of the street and its layout. (Experiences that remain truly novel for prolonged periods of time are such because we find no conception under which they fall, either immediately or upon reflection.)[16] In this way, our concepts and beliefs function to give meaning to our experiences. But by this account, we are not saying much that differs greatly from the principlist.

However, a terrible mistake is made when we take any of our concepts and beliefs as fixed, necessary, or a priori. We misunderstand the nature of these concepts (or principles, if you will) when priority is given to them over individual experiences. There is nothing "indispensable" about any of our existing concepts. Our categories, concepts, and principles must also be evaluated in the process of inquiry. For what are our principles (personal, social, political, scientific, or ethical) but a relatively stable set of experientially developed habits? As such, they both move us to action and are themselves movable (or modifiable). Principles, as Dewey has said, "represent conditions which have been ascertained during the conduct of continued inquiry to be involved in its own successful pursuit. . . . [P]rinciples are generated in the very process of control of continued inquiry" (LW12, 19). Like Charles Peirce before him, Dewey calls these kinds of principles "guiding" or "leading" principles. "According to this view, every inferential conclusion that is drawn [that is, every result of inquiry] involves a habit (either by way of expressing it or initiating it) in the *organic* [that is, living and evolving] sense of habit, since life is impossible without ways of action sufficiently general to properly be called *habits*" (LW12, 19). These habits as they are investigated, formulated, and developed become the leading principles of future inquiry.[17]

Unlike the basic four principles of Beauchamp and Childress and the formal principles of Engelhardt, then, pragmatic principles arise out of our activities and are always subject to revision or expulsion as further inquiry progresses. They are not foundational in any necessary sense but are primarily functional/operational, for if our principles are acquired habits, this implies not that specific principles exist a priori, but that principles only arise from our once-considered reactions to empirical situations that have developed subsequently as the basis for certain tendencies toward further kinds of actions whenever particular kinds of situations arise. In this sense, habits themselves are always general, but must be responsive to particular situations. They are also, however, modifiable by the specifics of the situations that occur. For example, my habit of walking across the street in the University district of Seattle is general in its scope, for it stands in reserve to be put into play *whenever* I step on to University Avenue. But it is modified by a context in which a particular parking meter's physical presence restricts the ability of my habit of walking to function adequately. These principles and concepts give meaning to new experiences, and yet are themselves transformed by each new experience (this is the "organic" sense of which Dewey speaks). "[We try] to apply to every new experience whatever from [our] old experience[s] will help [us] understand [them], and as this process of constant assumption and experimentation is fulfilled and refuted by results, [our] conceptions get body and clearness" (MW6, 281). And he might have added that our conceptions themselves might also change through this process.

Rather than reifying principles and developing rational grounds for their necessity, we must focus on the purpose and function of a principle as habit. This requires that we be reflective about not only the situation at hand, but our own classifications, conceptions, and beliefs that we use to try to understand situations. As James said, "Every way of classifying a thing [or activity] is but a way of handling it for some particular purpose. Conceptions, 'kinds,' are teleological instruments. No abstract concept can be a valid substitute for a concrete reality except with reference to a particular interest in the conceiver" (James [1882] 1977, 321). Principles, concepts, classifications, and so forth, as embodied by each individual, are stimulants to act according to the presumed meaning of an experience—they are habits.

Let us take a moment to recall what habits are. Dewey, again, tells us: "[H]abits are arts. They involve skill of sensory and motor organs, cunning or craft, and objective materials. They assimilate objective energies, and eventuate in command of environment. They require order, discipline, and manifest technique" (MW14, 15–16). Habits bind together bodily control, rational ability, and the surrounding environment where each element contributes to its development and success. Even a physiological habit like "[w]alking implicates the ground as well as the legs; speech demands air and human companionship, an audience as well as vocal cords. . . . [H]abits are ways of incorporating and using the environment in which the latter has its say as surely as the former" (MW14, 15). Habits involve the context that surrounds their function; they help to manifest, and are themselves manifest in, a social condition. "[S]ince habits involve the support of environing conditions, a society or some specific group of fellow-men is always accessory before and after the fact" (MW14, 16). They implicate the community around us as they manifest themselves in ways unique to each individual who calls them forth. Habits arise out of conduct and develop character, involving physiological and cultural material. They are the results of inquiry while they themselves shape further investigations. They are neither permanent and fixed, nor merely transient. As James tells us in *The Principles of Psychology*, habits have plasticity whereby they are capable of adaptation and change while remaining relatively stable; they are "weak enough to yield to influence, but strong enough not to yield all at once" (James [1890] 1950, 105).

Principles as habits can support the process of understanding ethical problems by providing questions to ask and motivations to fulfill, but they cannot be distant from the process of ethical inquiry. They must arise from a given situation and be adaptable, malleable, even discardable. They help give meaning to activity, but they themselves are habits of action that depend on social factors for their own meaning. If these factors are not to be found in a given context, the principle cannot be applied, and to reduce all ethical medical encounters to the interplay of four or fewer "basic" principles is to limit the possibilities of ethical activity and to do a great disservice to the diversity of individuals, relationships, and encounters themselves. No principle can be applicable to every given situation a priori. Habits are plastic; they mutate and adapt (they evolve) with each new situation that puts them into play. Principles as habits come into play when the appropriate stimulant strikes, energizing our malleable habits. Accordingly, to say "this" concept or "that" principle is the same in one case as another is, in its details, ridiculous. And, as should be clear, "in its details" is where all ethical work gets done.

Given this account, Engelhardt's a priori formalism is clearly incapable of doing any real ethical work here since his position denies the ability of empirical experience to ground ethical inquiry. To give credit to Beauchamp and Childress, however, in their support of the bioethical principles, they avoid making concrete claims about the nature of principles. They do not claim a specific a priori status to principles, for they claim that these principles arise out of "common morality." Carefully, they attempt to ground their philosophy in "considered judgments," which (as the argument goes) we all have and are beyond question during any particular investigation. However, we discover two things: (1) no further justification for the importance of principles is given, and (2) once stated, there is no discussion of the ultimate contingency of the principles. That is, as mentioned earlier in the chapter, Beauchamp and Childress separate the inductive process of developing principles from the deductive activity of justifying ethical judgments based on those principles. "Kicking the ladder away," Beauchamp and Childress treat their principles as foundational.

It is important to point out that I am *not* arguing that we have no commitments or steady habits that we bring to the table; nor do I disagree in the usefulness of principles in moral deliberation. However, the *status* of these habits, commitments, or "considered judgments" and the principles they produce is to be questioned. These so-called "principles of bioethics" are taken by Beauchamp and Childress as true for any given ethical inquiry. They write as though there is no conceivable alternative to the "holding sway" of these principles in ethical activities among individuals. Therefore, they end up giving important ethical priority to their principles, a priority that loses sensitivity to particular situations and "difficult cases."

SOME IMPLICATIONS FOR ETHICAL MEDICINE

Beauchamp and Childress's principlism and Engelhardt's formalism provide, if not too clearly, accounts of ethical inquiry. These positions attempt to give direction to bioethical practice and approaches to ethical problems in medicine. However, as we have already put into question, these methods are thinly developed and empty of any useful content for everyday, practical situations. Both theories leave us wanting in regards to determining specific actions.

In light of the inadequacies of principlism and formalism with respect to everyday, practical matters, I offer, throughout this work, a positive, pragmatic approach to ethical inquiry that begins in everyday problems, not "beyond" them. The emptiness of experiential/empirical content for both parties is particularly troubling given that ethical problems are found not in the abstract but in the concrete. The very meaning of an ethical problem comes from the situation out of which it arises.

In order to determine whether or not amputating a foot is warranted, we do not first appeal to principles, but to the details of the situation. If the amputation is in response to a child's kicking his little sister, we would say that this punishment is too harsh. However, if it is in response to the invasion of gangrene, we would be less inclined to see this as a punishment. In fact, many (though not all) might see this as an important invasive, medical procedure that can save a person's life. And yet, there are cases like the one used by Jonsen, Siegler, and Winslade (1992, 48–49), wherein a seventy-three-year-old patient refuses just such an amputation. Thus, the ability to determine the next step medically is completely wrapped up in the details: Why does the patient refuse? What does the patient want? What can health care professionals offer the patient? What are the reasons for wanting to perform the surgery? We are not here explicitly referring to and balancing abstract principles as much as we are beginning to recognize details that make a difference to our determined actions, and we cannot come to a final judgment concerning "the right thing to do" in either case without further investigation into the values and interests held by the participants in the situations.

To their credit, Beauchamp/Childress and Engelhardt are quite sensitive to the existence of others and the need for others to express their own desires. However, as we shall see in the next chapter, given the weaknesses in the moral frameworks of their arguments, their attempts to empower the other (in particular, a patient) through their uses of the principle of autonomy are inadequate and fall tragically short.

NOTES

1. Whereas the "principle of autonomy" is championed in both PBE 1979 and FB 1986, "respect for autonomy" is used in PBE 1994 and "permission" in FB 1996 as "updated" substitutions for the principle of autonomy.

2. This term was coined by Clouser and Gert (1990).

3. Anonymous, *Bulletin of Medical Ethics*, on the back cover of PBE 1994.

4. I will argue throughout this and the following chapter that though the authors do attempt changes in later editions designed to account for criticisms over the fifteen years since the first edition, the changes do not substantially affect the problems of principlism that I attack. Still other significant changes may appear in the fifth edition (2001), but that edition came out after this book went to press.

5. In the first edition, Beauchamp and Childress use the term "applied normative ethics" for their approach: "Our focus is *applied normative ethics*, because biomedical ethics is the application of general moral action-guides to biomedicine" (PBE 1979, 9). However, by the fourth edition, the authors deny that their approach is a case of "applied ethics": "The attempt to work out the implications of general theories for specific forms of conduct and moral judgment will be called *practical ethics* here, although it is often misleadingly called *applied ethics*" (PBE 1994, 4). However, since I see few *substantive* changes occur between 1979 and 1994, I see no reason to accept their later denial of "applied ethics" at face value.

6. Figures reflect March 2001 statistics. For the most current statistics see http://www.unos.org.

7. Cf. Clouser and Gert 1990.

8. Note that the idea of coherence used by Beauchamp and Childress is one of rational judgment to theory. This, then, should not be confused with the idea of coherence rendered from James's moral philosophy as described in chapter 1, where coherence concerns the invention of a unifying narrative that accounts for the expressed desires of ourselves *and* others. The difference, therefore, is between "coherence to a moral framework"—emphasis on theory—and "coherence of different experiences"—emphasis on praxis.

9. The "need" for a practice of specification is introduced in the fourth edition (PBE 1994) and does not appear in any of the earlier editions.

10. This is, itself, a highly questionable example given that the authors take for granted that, though any particular way of "specifying" these rules in order to perform a deceptive act on "moral grounds" may not itself by "justifiable," the deceiving act itself is better than covering the costs of medical technology through other means.

11. Allow me to make it clear that I do not fully subscribe to what is known as a "casuistic" approach advocated by Albert Jonsen and Steven Toulmin (1988). The problem with this approach is that certain simplified cases are treated as paradigms of ethical problems (cf. Jonsen, Siegler, and Winslade 1992). This approach to case-based ethics reduces to a form of ethics that looks much like principlism, where paradigmatic cases stand in for principles, more pluralistic, perhaps, but still highly problematic.

12. This "inadequacy" is the reason for the development of such apparatus as I discussed earlier—namely, "specifications." A clear retreat to the use of this apparatus can be seen in the following quote "[The principle of respect for autonomy] needs specification in particular contexts to become a practical guide to conduct, and appropriate specification will list valid exceptions" (PBE 1994, 126). Of course, this clearly begs questions such as, What is meant here by "appropriate"? and What would a "specification" of this principle look like?

13. Engelhardt believes that the four principles of Beauchamp and Childress are reducible to these two since the principle of autonomy requires that no harm come to a patient, and the principle of justice requires a "deserving" or broadly beneficial outcome.

14. This is an obviously Kantian reference to a necessary foundation that "transcends" any particular moral agent's viewpoint.

15. Cf. Loewy 1997 for a thorough critique of Engelhardt's narrow, bipolar sense of community.

16. One illustration of this can be found in the pop-culture movie *Phenomenon,* wherein there is an initially unexplained flash of light and subsequent intellectual enhancement of John Travolta's character.

17. See the previous chapter for a more thorough discussion of habits.

Chapter 3

Autonomy as Consent: An All-Too-Passive Concept

INTRODUCTION

The previous chapter attempted to explain the ethical positions of two different versions of bioethics at its "highest" level: the so-called principlism of Tom Beauchamp and James Childress on the one hand, and the formalism of H. Tristram Engelhardt on the other. I have argued that principlism as a framework in which moral deliberation should occur is inadequate to match the needs of particular problematic situations. Furthermore, though his formalism is decidedly different from principlism, Engelhardt's account of bioethical principles fares no better than Beauchamp and Childress's. Neither account is capable of meeting specific morally problematic events at the level of the particular problems that arise in the unique contexts that are always at play in each new situation. These inadequacies and weaknesses become even clearer when we investigate their respective accounts of the principle of autonomy.

The principles of autonomy—alternately known as autonomy, respect for autonomy, and permission[1]—as foundational or formal principles in these authors' theories are susceptible to the same general criticisms and dangers elaborated on in the previous discussion. However, the principle of autonomy in bioethics is taken by Beauchamp/Childress and Engelhardt as fundamental to both ethical activity and other bioethical principles, and thus merits special attention (cf. PBE 1994, 120; FB 1996, 108–9). Intended to provide and protect a space for individuals to express their desires and participate in situations that matter to them, the principle of autonomy has deep historical roots in Western culture, arising in the Enlightenment with authors as diverse as John Locke, Jean-Jacques Rousseau, and Immanuel Kant. The bioethical principle of autonomy clearly participates in and continues the Enlightenment emphasis on individualism and reason. Unfortunately, as we shall discuss in Alasdair MacIntyre's critique of Enlightenment autonomy, the bioethical emphasis on this principle proves to be incapable of empowering moral agents as it leaves the concept of the self empty and powerless. And this is particularly tragic in the medical setting where already dis-empowered patients seek to regain health in an attempt to participate in living. As I shall argue, contrary to the opinions of these authors, the principle of autonomy in bioethics does not adequately empower and is incapable of supporting active agency of the patient. Negatively, the principle does demand that constraints on moral activity be minimized, but the only positive aspect of the principle is surprisingly passive. As we shall see, though they obviously differ in how they get there, Beauchamp/Childress and Engelhardt arrive at the same place concerning the practical bearing of this principle in the concept of "informed consent," an idea that, though important in medicine, simply leaves the patient as patient—that is, passive—without promoting active participation by the patient in his or her own healing process, a participation that is essential for truly moral medical encounters.

BEAUCHAMP AND CHILDRESS: PRINCIPLE OF (RESPECT FOR) AUTONOMY

After explaining that their "account [of the principle of respect for autonomy] is essential to [their] objectives throughout subsequent chapters," Beauchamp and Childress define "autonomy" as "personal rule of the self that is free from both controlling interferences by others and from personal limitations that prevent meaningful choice, such as inadequate understanding" (PBE 1994, 120–21). Note that this definition attempts to make space for individual choice by implying that freedom consists in a lack of "controlling interferences" and "personal limitations." It is, on this account, a negative principle and clearly implies that control by others is a detriment to freedom.

They continue their account later: "We analyze autonomous action in terms of normal choosers who act (1) intentionally, (2) with understanding, and (3) without controlling influences that determine their action" (PBE 1994, 123). Intentionality, they claim, is not a matter of degree and is summed up as acting in such a way that the said action "correspond[s] to the agent's conception of how it was planned to be performed" (PBE 1994, 208). However, understanding and the absence of controlling influences do admit of degrees. That is, certain situations will allow us to understand and be controlled by others more or less depending on the case. For example, a patient in the early stages of Alzheimer's may be capable of comprehending physicians and others regarding her illness and treatment, but as the disease progresses, both understanding and the ability of the patient to act of her own accord diminishes. In these kinds of cases it is not uncommon nor is it typically troublesome to have others (family, physicians, and so on) make decisions with, for, and about such patients. For Beauchamp and Childress, this implies that "Actions therefore can be autonomous by degrees" (PBE 1994, 123), a revelation that leads them to the requirement that an action be "substantially autonomous." However, we are given no account of substantial autonomy since, as they correctly note, "appropriate criteria of substantial autonomy are best addressed in particular context, rather than pinpointed through a general theory" (PBE 1994, 124). Of course, we are then led back to our question of why they do not begin here with discussions of contexts rather than with general notions of autonomy itself.[2]

Noting at least one weakness themselves, by the fourth edition Beauchamp and Childress change from the principle of autonomy to the principle of respect for autonomy. They recognize that "Being autonomous is not the same as being respected as an autonomous agent" (PBE 1994, 125). It is the latter and not the former that must guide moral activities, and this principle "should not be used for persons who cannot act in a sufficiently autonomous manner"—that is, who cannot perform "substantially autonomous" actions. The principle is admittedly negative and is stated succinctly: "*Autonomous actions should not be subjected to controlling constraints by others*" (PBE 1994, 126). The principle obligates others to "stand clear" in the presence of substantially autonomous action.

Beauchamp and Childress go still further by interpreting their principle of respect for autonomy for practical purposes: "The basic paradigm of autonomy in health care, politics, and other contexts is *express* and informed consent" (PBE 1994, 128). Through some clear expression (either explicit, tacit, implied, or presumed), consent to, agreement for, or permission to perform actions that include the consenting agent is the practical exercise of autonomy, and making a space for that expression (or the omission of that consent) is the practice of respecting autonomy.

Thus, Beauchamp and Childress's account of the principle of autonomy begins as a negative expression concerning the need to minimize interference by others and ends in a practical (positive) expression that the principle of autonomy bear out in experience as "informed consent." Of course, we are left with several significant concerns such as, What constitutes a "controlling influence"? Who or what determines "substantial autonomy" in any given situation? And most important, How can the passive notion of "consent" help empower patients in the numerous different medical encounters in which they find themselves struggling to regain healthy living?

As with their account of the basic biomedical principles generally, Beauchamp and Childress's take on the principle of autonomy leaves us with important questions unanswered, and I turn now to see if Engelhardt's account fares any better.

ENGELHARDT: PRINCIPLE OF AUTONOMY (OR PERMISSION)

The Kantian influence on Engelhardt is most recognizable in his development of the principle of autonomy. As we have already discussed, Engelhardt believes this principle to be the necessary formal condition for the possibility of moral activity. Like Kant, Engelhardt's principle of autonomy has no empirical content, but provides the basis for ethical social interaction. This account implies (as with Kantian theory as well) that autonomous agents as rational beings somehow have full moral capabilities, if not content, prior to their existential interactions, and since (as we know from Kant) any existential interaction can interfere with freedom, the principle of autonomy has little value. More precisely, it is of no value at all, either negative or positive, but instead provides the possibility for value through the principle of beneficence.

For Engelhardt, the principle of autonomy is not itself authoritative; that is, it does not have power to determine action. It does, however, provide for "authority in action." It states, "Authority for actions involving others in a secular pluralistic society is derived from the free and informed consent of those involved" (FB 1996, 124; FB 1986, 85). In other words, the principle of autonomy is the basis for authorizing actions toward others by expressing one all-important necessary formal condition: In order for moral activity to occur in medicine, permission must be sought by the physician and given by the patient. Though derived from formal considerations, surprisingly Engelhardt's reduction of the principle of autonomy in practice to "informed consent" is, for all intents and purposes, no different than Beauchamp and Childress before him. As a basis for moral activity, Engelhardt's principle (like that of Beauchamp and Childress) does little to promote active participation of the patient in his or her own healing process, and as I will show in the following chapters, this lack of empowering patients and engaging them in their own health care cuts off the possibility for meaningful interactions and does a great disservice to selves as a social product.

MACINTYRE ON ENLIGHTENMENT AUTONOMY

Before moving to a positive account of the self, it may behoove us to take one more moment to reflect on the weaknesses of the aforementioned principles of autonomy, for a thorough understanding of the weaknesses will help put my own position into stronger relief. As it has been mentioned above, the principle of autonomy in any of the previously discussed forms stems from its acceptance of Enlightenment individualism that takes the self as insular and atomic, fundamentally cut off from society. This Enlightenment ideal self has been roundly criticized by many philosophers. Particularly within the last two decades, it has been assaulted by so-called communitarians.

Communitarians take the nature of the self, as expressed by Enlightenment-type autonomy theorists (that is, classical liberals) to be a false account. Whereas the classical liberal believes selves are, in their true essence, fully formed prior to the social relations with which they later become bound, and further that these very relations among selves and between individuals and communities are hindrances to the truly free self, the communitarian sees no way to divide selves from their relations without losing the very meaning of selfhood. For the communitarian, selves are essentially tied to the social contexts in which they are a part. As I have said, this communitarian critique has been raised by several philosophers in the last twenty years—for example, Michael Sandel, Martha Nussbaum, and Charles Taylor—but none more directly and successfully than MacIntyre.

In his well-known work *After Virtue*, MacIntyre argues for a neo-Aristotelian take on ethics with its focus on character and telos. His position is set in stark contrast to twentieth-century "emotivism," which, in MacIntyre's account, has its historical roots in and takes its cues from the modernist Enlightenment project of the seventeenth, eighteenth, and even nineteenth centuries as manifested in philosophers from Germany to the British Isles. The Enlightenment project of justifying morality, in MacIntyre's view, breaks down, and "provided the historical background against which the predicaments of our own culture can become intelligible" (MacIntyre 1984, 39). Though MacIntyre has his own positive (Aristotelian) agenda to pursue, it is his negative criticism of the Enlightenment project and its take on the autonomous self that most concerns me here, for his assault on Enlightenment autonomy holds equally for the contemporary bioethical principle of autonomy as espoused by Beauchamp/Childress and Engelhardt.[3]

In chapter 4 of *After Virtue*, MacIntyre describes the historical roots of the failure of modern Western moralists from David Hume to Kant to Søren Kierkegaard as the attempt to ground morality based on rational argument, either negative or positive. He explains that Kierkegaard's ethical subject is directly in line with Kantian morality, a morality based on the universal power and scope of reason, while Hume's "ethics as passion" remains both conservative and inconsistent. Hume's moral theory accepts normative values while concurrently devising rational (negative) arguments *against* the power of reason to ground morality. Thus, the major players in Enlightenment moral philosophy all look to reason, in a universal sense, as the basis for ethical injunctions.

MacIntyre then goes on to show in chapter 5 why this Enlightenment project fails. Beginning with the notion that "there is a fundamental contrast between man-as-he-happens-to-be and man-as-he-could-be-if-he-realized-his-essential-nature," he states, "Ethics is the science which is to enable men to understand how they make the transition from the former state to the latter" (MacIntyre 1984, 52). However, modern secular philosophy's "rejection" of the "teleological" part of the "essential"[4] human nature equation leaves only rules of action (leading to what end?) and "a certain view of untutored-human-nature-as-it-is" (MacIntyre 1984, 55). Morality thus becomes a move back to original human nature rather than a move toward a potential character. MacIntyre analyzes this move in terms of a loss of the "functional" concept of human being or self.

[A]ccording to [ancient Greek] tradition to be a man is to fill a set of roles each of which has its own point and purpose: member of family, citizen, soldier, philosopher, servant of God. It is only when man is thought of as an individual prior to and apart from all roles that "man" ceases to be a functional concept. (MacIntyre 1984, 59)

MacIntyre clearly accepts the ancient Greek view, lamenting its loss in modernist accounts of morality and the self. The loss comes from no longer viewing the concept of the self as constitutively relational in character, always-already in and defined by the communities in which it takes part.

MacIntyre continues, "What I have described in terms of a loss of traditional structure and content was seen by the most articulate of [the Enlightenment's] philosophical spokesmen as the achievement of the self of its proper autonomy" (MacIntyre 1984, 60). Enlightenment philosophers, then, understood their position to entail a radical and fundamental achievement, "liberation" of the self from the social bonds that inhibited free movement and expression. On this level, their theories *are* revolutionary. The Enlightenment emphasis on liberation and individuality does succeed as a negative critique of the prevailing political and social order of the time. As John Dewey also points out, "The heralds of this [liberal] gospel were acutely conscious of the evils of the social estate in which they found themselves" (MW9, 98). And, still later in another work, Dewey continues, "The ideas of [the Enlightenment] . . . were potent in criticism and in analysis. They released forces that had been held in check" (LW11, 23). However, this "gospel" of individualism in the Enlightenment, though "potent" in the negative, had no "positive" powers for focusing activity. Dewey reminds us, "[A]nalysis is not construction, and release of force does not itself give direction to the force that is set free" (LW11, 23).

Both MacIntyre and Dewey clearly and decisively reject the Enlightenment account of this self, for it leaves the self as contentless, empty of power, and at odds with its own experience. Enlightenment concepts of autonomy developed frustrations for moral deliberation that continue today.

> Contemporary moral experience . . . has a paradoxical character. For each of us is taught to see himself or herself as an autonomous agent; but each of us also becomes engaged by modes of practice . . . which involve us in manipulative relationships with others. Seeking to protect the autonomy that we have learned to prize, we aspire ourselves *not* to be manipulated by others; seeking to incarnate our own principles and stand-point in the world of practice, we find no way open to us to do so except by directing towards others those very manipulative modes of relationship which each of us aspires to resist in our own case. The incoherence of our attitudes and our experience arises from the incoherent conceptual scheme which we have inherited. (MacIntyre 1984, 68)

Enlightenment-based autonomy leaves us fundamentally divided from, and therefore at odds with, others as we seek to exercise control of the environment we find ourselves in—an environment that includes other autonomous individuals. And these theories give us no recourse for moral deliberation. As MacIntyre argues, the formal nature of the Enlightenment self can do no better than yield arbitrary choice because there is no positive account for constructive activity. The self as "autonomous" is empty and void of empirical content; as such, choice and motive are fundamentally divided from the actions that ensue. According to the Enlightenment theorists, choice and motive in moral conduct are moments of reason, not of action, but somehow (and paradoxically) they cause the actions that follow. The fault here lies precisely in the loss of a functional concept of self that is defined in its relation to others and the environment at large, for this functional concept of self shows that moral choice is neither drawn from the dictates of pure reason and motivations of a "good will" nor can it arise prior to acting within existential situations. Selves as functional are in processes of moral deliberation and choice; that is, choice is action. Motive and choice are "not then a drive *to* action, or something which moves *to* doing something. [They *are*] the movement of the self as a whole" (LW7, 291).

MacIntyre continues his book, arriving at a positive position on the self wrapped up in the concept of narrative (to which I will return in the next chapter), and his own positive account of ethics, based on Aristotelian philosophy. Surprisingly, however, MacIntyre's appreciation of the functional character of the concept of self takes no cues from the highly influential turn-of-the-century movement in psychology known as "functionalism." This movement grew out of pragmatism as a psychological account of the self that, like MacIntyre, sees the self as a functional concept always-already tied up in relationships. Both William James and Dewey did much to develop and expand this "school" of thought, but it is the social psychology of George Herbert Mead, Dewey's colleague at the University of Chicago, that most thoroughly (if not always clearly) explains the functional self as a product of social relationships in community.

WHERE TO GO FROM HERE

There should be no surprise that bioethics in the hands of the authors we have been discussing has placed priority on the principle of autonomy. Western culture itself, especially since the Enlightenment, has championed the autonomous individual as the focal point of moral activity. The language of autonomy is *our* language. It is supported in theory and practice in academia, medicine, and society. However, the notion of the atomic self that undergirds these theories fundamentally misunderstands the nature of the self, which, as I will argue in the subsequent chapters, is not prior and opposed to society or "the other," but instead is socially situated and socially constructed. This basic Enlightenment misunderstanding of the self carries through to contemporary bioethics and leads to principles of autonomy that have little moral power in the face of actual existential situations calling for moral deliberation.

Although the communitarian critique of Enlightenment autonomy by people like MacIntyre is quite powerful in calling attention to inadequacies of the classical liberal theorists, it is not itself complete. In particular, the communitarian position does not respond sufficiently to concerns of oppression by the majority and complete sublimation of individuality by community interests.

In the following chapter, I will turn to Mead's understanding of the socially situated self in an attempt to give a more thorough account of selves and communities, which does justice to the communitarian critique and furthers insights of selves and communities to avoid standard criticisms of communitarianism itself. However, what we can say quite emphatically to this point is that the principle of autonomy, in the theories of Beauchamp/Childress and Engelhardt, is both negative and passive in its practical bearings, leaving the patient as "patient," disempowered except through her ability to consent to be worked upon by others. If we, instead, wish to empower patient and professional agency and participation in medical encounters, it is clear that we are in need of a more substantial and richer theory of the self and a reconstruction of, or substitution for, the idea of autonomy itself.

NOTES

1. "The principle of autonomy" is the phrase used by Beauchamp/Childress and Engelhardt in the first editions of their books. However, by the fourth edition of *Principles of Biomedical Ethics*, Beauchamp and Childress begin to use the phrase "the principle of respect for autonomy," and Engelhardt, in the second edition of *The Foundations of Bioethics*, uses the term "the principle of permission." However, in both cases, neither account differs substantially from previous editions. Therefore, without desiring to ignore any possibly important differences, I shall hereafter use the term "the principle of autonomy" to refer to all three of these different manifestations of what I argue are the same practical idea.

2. See the discussion in the previous chapter concerning the question of why Beauchamp and Childress begin with principles when they consistently admit that they are unable to give aid in specific cases and contexts.

3. Though MacIntyre himself would eschew such comparisons, his criticisms and insights into Enlightenment moral theories have a great deal in common with analogous discussions of empiricism and rationalism by pragmatist authors like Dewey, and thus fits quite well with the focus of my project.

4. There is a deeply rooted Aristotelian conception of static, purposeful human nature in MacIntyre's work that is not endorsable by the evolutionary, antifoundational character of pragmatism. This, albeit metaphysically important, difference does not detract from the main critical thrust of his discussion of Enlightenment theories.

Chapter 4

Self as Situated Social Product: The Functionality of Narratives

INTRODUCTION

I have just argued that the use of bioethical principles in general, and the principle of autonomy in particular, falls importantly and tragically short as a tool to empower individuals in medical encounters. Though the principle of autonomy does attempt to clear a space for individual choice, it does not and cannot promote active agency, and relies instead on the useful but far too limited notion of "informed consent." This principle, in its promoted form, is surprisingly empty of moral content and only minimally helpful in most medical situations. Autonomy, as has been alluded to earlier, is the brainchild of Enlightenment individualism, which takes the self to be prior to any of its social relations. However, as Alasdair MacIntyre has shown, it is this supposed insularity of the individual when in her free state that is the fundamental problem with the principle of autonomy.

The current chapter will attempt to reconstruct our notion of the self, not as an isolated entity, but as a product and process of social interaction and community. This reconstruction will leave behind the too-thin idea of the insular individual, but it will not lose individuality. Though a person intimately integrates with the social structures in which she develops, the individual is not subsumed under or consumed by them. Obviously, individuals are distinguishable from each other, but further, "there is not merely difference or distinction [between individuals], but something unique or irreplaceable in value, an unique difference of value" (MW15, 170). This value is not intrinsic (as in, for example, Kant's theory), but is developed, contingent, and ever changing through the social interactions in which individuals participate. My alternative to autonomy theory offers a positive hope for future work in medical ethics. It replaces the classical notion of the atomic self with a conception of self as mediated through narrative and, thereby, community.

I take the concept of the self to be not denoting some entity or substance but as a functional distinction that emphasizes and arises from specific occurrences, aspects, and processes in experience. It is impossible fundamentally to set the individual self as over-and-against society; each of us is inextricably developed by and developing of community itself. This leaves the idea of the insular individual behind and allows for new understandings about the moral life to prevail, both in and out of medical encounters.

I begin my discussion with George Herbert Mead's social psychology in order to develop an altogether different notion of the self as a product of social interaction in community. I am aided in this endeavor by concepts of "narrative," by which I mean nothing more than the "stories we tell," both about ourselves and others, not fictions but life stories of individuals, communities, and even cultures that are used to make sense of and bring meaning to living in the world. As we shall see, this functional application of what I call narrative significance implicates a context and implies the presence and influence of others.

The self is a product of community, while at the same time, reflexively helping to produce the communities of which it is a part. Of course, this understanding of the self demands a rendering of what community itself is, and this will be a focus midway through the chapter. Furthermore, the implications of these insights for medical encounters will be taken up in greater detail in the following chapter.

MEAD AND THE SELF AS SOCIAL PRODUCT

During the last decade of the nineteenth century and the first three decades of the twentieth, Mead crafted his insightful philosophical psychology of social behaviorism. Influenced by William James's landmark work, *The Principles of Psychology*, John Dewey's writings in functional psychology, and Alfred North Whitehead's process philosophy, Mead determined, like James before him, that the self is not an entity prior to social relations, but instead comes to be in and because of social processes. Recognized primarily in sociological circles, Mead's writings (most posthumously edited from lecture notes) have gone largely unnoticed by philosophers and psychologists. However, it is this relatively unknown and rather dense material that I wish to explore in order to elucidate the following claim: "[M]inds and selves are essentially social products, products of phenomena of the social side of human experience" (Mead [1934] 1962, 1).

Mead's psychology explains that what we call the "self," rather than being an entity upon which attributes and relations are "hung," is actually an organized complex of attitudes that reflexively implicates both the individual and society. Certainly, biological, organic individuals are uniquely situated in and created out of complex biological processes. That is, at birth (or conception, if you wish—there is no need to argue this point here), the infant starts as a mass of cells and biochemical activities. However, this organic individual should not be mistaken for a "self"; she is no *self* at all. The newborn makes no immediate distinctions between her body or needs and the movements of the environment of which she is a part. The thumb is not *her* thumb; it is an object that appears, then satisfies, in a matter wholly foreign to the child. In this way the child *undergoes* experience but does not comprehend or control it.

The *self*, on the other hand, is a conscious, interacting being in the world—a responsible and reflective character. The self makes distinctions and is conscious of its place in the world relative to its environment. However, these qualities do not and cannot arise until interactions with others occur. Through these interactions, the individual organism (usually in the form of a baby or young child) begins to recognize and respond to others. At first, the child simply plays games that mirror the actions of others, taking on roles and characters, merely imitating what she sees. Children smile at our smiles, laugh because we laugh, touch what we touch. Even later, this continues as they dress in our clothes, play with our tools, and speak in affected voices because that is what they see and hear.

However, slowly, individuals creatively separate the actions of others from their own. Rather than parroting others' actions, individuals look for responses from others to their own actions. Dogs growl and bare their teeth; children blurt out a noise. Mead calls these actions "gestures," and gestures gain their own meaning by the responses others have to them. The dog's growl *signifies nothing unless* we act scared because of it. The baby's cry means that it is time to change the diaper, not because of the infant's *intent*, but because of the parent's (or caregiver's) *response*.[1] The broken glass has no meaning to the child until an adult scolds her for breaking it; at that point, the broken glass *signifies* "trouble."

Soon, the young individual becomes aware of the attitudes of others to the extent that she begins anticipating those attitudes in selecting gestures appropriate to the situation. This activity develops quickly into the use of what Mead calls "significant symbols" where the individual in making the gesture anticipates the response in others. Mead states, "Gestures become significant symbols when they implicitly arouse in the individual making them the same responses which they explicitly arouse, or are supposed to arouse, in other individuals, the individuals to whom they are addressed" (Mead [1930] 1962, 47). These "significant symbols" most often come in the form of "vocal gestures"—that is, language. Language, and all other significant symbols for that matter, objectifies within the conversation the individual who is speaking; it treats her as an object to her*self*. Thus, the self first comes to be *reflexively*. The child says "bottle" in anticipation of the response by the parent to hand over the nippled object. But in saying "bottle," the child reacts to the object (if only internally) in the same way as the parents are expected to react. The child leans toward it, reaches for it, and becomes as much a member of the audience as the parents do, that is, by listening to her*self*.

The self arises, then, in "self-conscious" behavior that objectifies the self to itself. This objectifying move incorporates an awareness of the attitudes of the other. More specifically, it takes on the attitude of the community itself, or, in

Mead's language, the "generalized other." "The organized community or social group which gives to the individual his unity of self may be called the 'generalized other.' The attitude of the generalized other is the attitude of the whole community" (Mead [1934] 1962, 154). The self, then, arises by way of an awareness and an internalizing of the "attitudes" of the communities of which we are a part. Thus, Mead states, "In this way every gesture comes within a given social group or community to stand for a particular act or response, namely, the act or response which it calls forth explicitly in the individual who makes it" (Mead [1934] 1962, 47). (I will return to the idea of "community" later.)

The implications for the concept of "self," here, are obvious. Mead does not accept the prevailing modernist view of a prior self whose originary being comes fully formed. Instead, he takes the self to be the product of social interaction. But even this is misleading, for there is no "one" self, but,

> We divide ourselves up in all sorts of different selves with reference to our acquaintances. We discuss politics with one and religion with another. There are all sorts of selves answering to all sorts of different social reactions. It is the social process itself that is responsible for the appearance of the self; it is not there as a self apart from this type of experience. . . . There is usually an organization of the whole self with reference to the community to which we belong, and the situation in which we find ourselves. (Mead [1934] 1962, 142–43)

Community, then, is constitutive of and prior to the self. "It cannot be said that the individuals come first and the community later, for the individuals arise in the very process [of living] itself" (Mead [1934] 1962, 189). It is the taking on of community attitudes that make us "who we are" in any important sense.

> This getting of the broad activities of any given social whole or organized society as such within the experiential field of any one of the individuals involved or included in that whole is, in other words, the essential basis and prerequisite of the fullest development of that individual's self. (Mead [1934] 1962, 155)

Finally, this organization of the self has important moral consequences, for gestures of any significance must recognize and respond to others as we take on their attitudes as our own. And the meaning of our actions come, not by way of our intentions (though they may arise from our own impulses), but in how they are taken by others—that is, how they bear out in their consequences.

> If we look now towards the end of the action rather than toward the impulse itself, we find that those ends are good which lead to the realization of the self as a social being. *Our morality gathers about our social conduct. It is as social beings that we are moral beings.* On the one side stands the society which makes the self possible, and on the other side stands the self that makes a highly organized society possible. The two answer to each other in moral conduct. (Mead [1934] 1962, 386 [emphasis mine])

Moral activity occurs among social beings aware of this social self. Moral conduct and judgments must themselves be social such that "one can never [judge] simply from his own point of view. *We have to look at it from the point of view of a social situation.* . . . The only rule that an ethics can present is that an individual should rationally [and imaginatively] deal with all the values that are found in a specific problem" (Mead [1934] 1962, 387–88 [emphasis mine]). This is Mead's version of James's admonition to "invent some manner" of satisfying the demands of others and of Dewey's "moral artistry" (see chapter 1), all three of which move beyond Enlightenment individualism by accepting a social, "functional" nature to the concept of self. In other words, since my activities are never exclusively my own—that is, they arise, in part, from the social conditions in which I find myself and will consequently affect others of my social group—if I wish to perform my actions "to the good," I must account for the many (and often competing) interests at play in the situation. Those interests arise from other selves who are part of the environment in which I wish to exercise my own (communally constituted) desires. As Dewey has said, it is not that morality *ought* to be social; "morality is social."

COMMUNITY IN SELVES, COMMUNITY OF SELVES[2]

Mead's self arises in the very process of organic community, and this community is defined in terms of Mead's "generalized other" that is both a dispositional (or "perspectival") and an ideal (or "normative") sense of community in which there is an awareness among individuals that their interests are best satisfied in and through the satisfaction of others' desires.[3] In community, members share in what Justus Buchler calls a "potency for many individuals" of a given situation, event, or object.[4] They are "moved" by the same things, taking similar attitudes towards objects of beauty, enjoyment of sport, and appreciation of foods, among others. But further still, there is a normative element in communities that establishes an organized way of behaving such as language use and social roles. All this eventuates in an ideal, "democratic" life where individual differences are taken seriously by others while coming together for a common good because of our shared attitudes using normative standards in language and so on. As Beth Singer puts it, "The condition of community is one of sameness-in-difference, of partial commonality of perspective among persons whose perspectives as individuals also include other perspectives, some unique to themselves and some shared with members of multiple communities to which they belong" (Singer 1995, 4).[5]

One explanation of this idea(l) of community comes from Dewey when he says, "The parts of a machine work with a maximum of coöperativeness for a common result, but they do not form a community. If, however, they were all cognizant of the common end and all interested in it so that they regulate their specific activity in view of it, then they would form a community" (MW9, 8). The contrast highlighted by Dewey's illustration is that between a mere gathering of individuals and a community. The individual members of a gathering work toward their own ends, which, by either chance or external construction of the situation, may or may not fit well with the ends of others in the group. The coworkers (nurses, specialists, and subspecialists) in a hospital, for instance, can easily find themselves members of a "mere" social gathering in their daily activities to the extent that their activities are routinized and their pursuits of ends are limited to their individual tasks. These bonds are strengthened to form a community, however, when individuals become aware of the ends of others, take others' ends as common and shared, and recognize that satisfying the interests of others in the community is of value to themselves. Members of a community, while attempting to fulfill their own interests, take note of others' desires and adjust and regulate their activities and employ means appropriate to the mutual fulfillment of common ends. This awareness of mutually fulfilling interests manifests itself through a sharing of activities—through truly shared experiences where a common perspective is forged—and responsibilities in order to consummate the desires of all members of the community.[6]

This is most important because an integration of interests and the awareness of this integration ("awareness," here, being an active process of regulating and adjusting activity) yields the very experience *of* community. Culturally, this amounts to individual and social interests being satisfied simultaneously; that is, our activities satisfy both our individual desires and community interests, and vice versa. I would venture to say that this is precisely what happens in a well-run emergency room, staffed by professionals who know and trust each other. As a flurry of activity arises, all participants in the care of an emergent patient, though given particular roles (attending, lead, nursing support, etc.), are encouraged to view their activities not simply from a narrow personal perspective but from the shared perspective of affecting a good final goal—namely, the best care for this particular patient.

For another, not directly medical example, we can, following Mead, turn to baseball where, for example, the shortstop on the team has certain tasks to perform on the field, ends that she desires to satisfy—namely, fielding the ball between second and third, as well as covering "the bag" for some throws, and so on.[7] But these tasks are regulated by the actions of the others on the team and the understanding by the shortstop as to how others' actions affect her own—for example, the shortstop must cover third on a bunt down the line and a runner on second. As a matter of fact, her very position exists only within the complex of the game, the other players, and the rules they all follow.

It must be clearly noted, though, that regulating individual activity according to community demands need not wholly subsume individual interests under community ones.

[E]very individual is in his own way unique. Each one experiences life from a different angle than anybody else, and consequently has something distinctive to give others. . . . Each individual . . . is a new beginning; the universe itself is, as it were, taking a fresh start in him and trying to do something, even if on a small scale, that it has never done before. (LW5, 127)

Each of us, then, contributes uniquely to the community in a way that would be altogether lost to the community if that particular individual were not present.

For example, situated within the domain of the game of baseball, the shortstop has a broad range in which to pursue her own individual ends with her own individual style (such as hitting well, fielding spectacularly, becoming a star, and so on—for example, nobody plays the game like Alex Rodriguez) while contributing to the common ends of the team of which she is a part. In the case of a group of baseball players such as the Seattle Mariners, this community is fundamentally different with the contributions of Rodriguez than without, and now that he has moved on to the Texas Rangers, the team will be affected in noticeable ways that require adjustments by the other players.[8] Further, the unique contributions of all the players add not only to fulfilling their own personal desires to play the game well but to get the Mariners into the playoffs and beyond.

The key, then, in positive, progressive human interaction, it would seem, is to balance individual and social interests by finding ways to retain individual desires and values (in their vast multiplicity and diversity) while making them work within the social good.[9] As Dewey points out, this is an idea as old as Plato, but unlike the ancient Greek view that divided humans into only three rigid categories, Dewey stresses that there are as many categories as there are humans.

We cannot better Plato's conviction that an individual is happy and society well organized when each individual engages in those activities for which he has a natural equipment. . . . But progress in knowledge has made us aware of the superficiality of Plato's lumping of individuals and their original powers into a few sharply marked-off classes; it has taught us that original capacities are indefinitely numerous and variable. (MW9, 96)

To develop a Deweyan democratic community, then, in this radical plurality requires "utilization of the specific and variable qualities of individuals," an emphasis that promotes individual intelligence within existing and ever-changing biological and cultural matrices (MW9, 97). But still further, it takes an educated ability continuously to locate oneself within a community of one's choosing. The ideal here, as we have seen in the above examples, is a community of individual interests that work together so that individual and social ends are contemporaneous (or coincident) and inclusive of each other.

Of course, the ideal is difficult to obtain. Communal associations often take complex negotiations and require well-stated arguments. These are not always pleasant and are rarely neat or clean. There are a vast array of factors that must be accounted for, factors that arise in the experiences of individuals and groups. (For example, Carol Gilligan's famous work [1993] on the psychological and moral experiences of women demonstrates just one among many issues that should be taken serious in our community-building processes.[10]) But so long as negotiations both account for the interest of all participants and accomplish some end that envelops those interests to the highest degree possible given the circumstances, a community of shared experience will arise. Community is found in a "society that makes provision for *participation in its good of all its members on equal terms* and which secures flexible readjustments of its institutions through interaction of the different forms of associated life" (MW9, 105 [emphasis mine]). And members of such a community will find that their own "[s]ocial perceptions and interests can be developed only in a genuinely social medium—one where there is give and take in the building up of a common experience" (MW9, 368).

We see, then, that Dewey and Mead agree; community makes selves and selves make up community.

> Human society as we know it could not exist without minds and selves, since all its most characteristic features presuppose the possession of minds and selves by its individual members; but its individual members would not possess minds and selves if these had not arisen within or emerged out of the human social process in its lower stages of development. (Mead [1934] 1962, 227)

Furthermore, they also agree that accounting for all interests at play in the community is an important part of acting within (as part of) a community.

NARRATIVE AND THE SOCIAL SELF

Mead's own explanation of language as "significant symbol" makes clear that social selves communicate by way of "dramatically rehearsing" (in any number of conscious and unconscious ways) the attitude of the communities that surround them. And as Steve Fesmire (recall chapter 1) explains, this imaginative projection of community attitudes by selves is often a "story-structured" capacity that guides our conduct and develops our selves (Fesmire 1995). This "story-structured" process I will call "narrative," and I wish to argue that given his account of the process of how selves come to be, Mead's social, functional self could also be termed a "narrative self"—that is, a unique nexus of social attitudes that come together through the stories we enact and tell about ourselves and others.

Selves are constructs, built, in part, through the comings and goings within a community. One way to understand these interactions of selves is through narrative accounts. We can and do construct and use stories to make sense of our experiences, and this use of stories can be valuable to investigate.[11]

First, narratives do not begin from nothing. They start where we are now, using both past and present situations.[12] We weave a story that, in part, takes account of certain "facts" of life. These facts are interpretations of events involving people, places, and things. In their very use, these facts are considered "relevant," and "relevant" facts are choices made by individuals revealing how and where they stand now. In this way, narratives are purposive. They are told for some reason(s). Stories about ourselves and others weave the pieces of experience into a complex fabric. Thus, stories do more than recount the past or explain the present; they also project into the future. Personal and social narratives are taken up into experience that is itself future-directed. Imaginative projection places history into the context of the ever-evolving self and the constantly changing community environment.

But still further, our stories are made not simply in our tellings but through our activities. When asked to explain who we are, we speak, and when attempting to express who we are, we simply act. We are not merely storytellers but narrative actors. We enact the stories that are our lives in the very processes of living. Narratives are a means by which we create lives that give meaning to ourselves and others.

Given their uses of experience and pursuits of meaning, we can see that every narrative functions in at least two ways—one descriptive and another creative—which are not wholly separable.

Creative Description

As description, a narrative recalls "facts" of life and culture. It highlights features of experience that are available (or are now made available) to all. Description for this reason is often considered to be "objective." This label must be used with caution, however, since no subject/object distinction exists in experience prior to a narrative and its purpose. As James points out, *"Experience, I believe, has no such inner duplicity; and the separation of it into . . .* [subject/object] *comes, not by way of subtraction, but by way of addition*—the addition, to a given concrete piece of it, of other sets of experiences, in connection with which severally its use or function may be of two different kinds" (James [1904] 1977, 172 [James's emphasis]). A specific narrative adds to experience through the use of other narratives in order to create functional distinctions like subject/object. Once this reflective story is developed, the description is as "objective" for the members of a community as any "fact" can be since it is open to observation and exploration by anyone.

However, there is another "objectification" that occurs that is also important. Stories told by an individual about (some aspect[s] of) that individual "objectify" the self to itself. That is, the narrator in creating the story makes it available in an "objective," observable form not only to others but to herself as well. As we have seen, Mead discusses this nicely in his account of the "genesis of the self." Mead claims that we come to self-consciousness, and self-evaluation, by way of language, or what he calls "vocal gestures." We narrate our life stories always in some common language. Language is always-already social and, thus, causes the speaker "to act toward himself as the other acts toward him" (Mead [1932] 1980, 189). Language objectifies the self to itself by situating the self within a community. Mead, thus, concludes that the self, by way of the narratives it tells about it-self, is socially constructed.

David Burrell and Stanley Hauerwas echo this in their discussion of narrative when they say,

> The language the agent uses to describe his behavior, to himself and to others, is not uniquely his; it is *ours*. . . . An agent cannot make his behavior mean anything he wants, since at the very least it must make sense within his own story, as well as be compatible with the narrative embodied in the language he uses. (Burrell and Hauerwas 1979, 168)

To be a story, it must "make sense" in some way. Even if someone could mean any-thing she wants, this "wanting" is itself a function of *available* descriptions—for example, no one in the Middle Ages could *want* to play major league baseball or use MRIs to diagnose anatomical structures. As said above, narratives begin where we are, and thus arise as part of an epoch and community in which they originate (which is not to say that they might not *later* transcend that epoch or community).

Selves can live in isolation from others and dream as they want at various times in their lives, but even their dreams begin in what they know—namely, their com-munities. "*After* a self has arisen, it in a certain sense provides for itself its own social experiences, and so we can conceive of an absolutely solitary self. But *it is impossible* to conceive of a self *arising* outside of social experience" (Mead [1934] 1962, 140 [emphasis mine]). And, again, Burrell and Hauerwas state, "The fact is that the first person singular is seldom the assertion of the solitary 'I,' but rather the narrative of the I" (Burrell and Hauerwas 1979, 168). The "narra-tive I" is the "I" that is expressed in actions, through words, and always is a re-sult of community attitudes uniquely taken up and developed further by the indi-vidual. Language is never simply mine alone; even in introspective moments, I "talk" to myself using the language given to me by the community through which I have become enculturated. Through the process of communication with others (or through the medium of the other), a meaningful self is produced.

If we accept this, we must also accept that autonomy as independence from the other is an illusion. Selves are only in relation to others, and yet "autonomy" finds its natural home in the Enlightenment notion of the self as insular and antecedent to community. "Autonomy," in this classical sense, fundamentally misunder-stands selves. We may be able to use the term in some colloquial way, but philo-sophical discussions of autonomy from Locke to Engelhardt do not escape the Enlightenment view of the self, and thus, they define "autonomy" in an essen-tially negative fashion as the self devoid of *restrictive* social relationships.[13] However, the "narrative" insights that I have just brought out show the self as me-diated, as a social product. This does not mean that we lose the individual; we re-construct it. As Dewey has pointed out, "individualism" has run its course, but in-dividuality still holds sway (cf. LW5, 41–124). To be an individual is to be a particular socially located self, and to respect such an individual is to facilitate and enhance the particular social interactions that constitute that self. These interactions occur within communities of selves, and the selves are, in turn, shaped by these communities.

The arising of the self implicates community and does so through the language and other communications we use. It has been here described as a narrative process of locating oneself within her community that, in turn, fashions anew the self attempting to be located. The production of the self by way of community through narratives leads us to the second aspect of stories—the creative.

Descriptive Creation

Narrative as creation weaves new patterns out of and into old ones. It takes available subject matter and attempts to make a coherent account of it for oneself or another; as J. M. Bernstein writes,

> One of the ways human beings assess and interpret the events of their life [*sic*] is through the *construction of plausible narratives.* Narratives represent events not as general laws but rather as elements of a history where a continuing individual or collective subject suffers or brings about dramatic, i.e. meaningful, changes. A change is meaningful in relation to past *and future events.* (Bernstein 1990, 55 [emphasis mine])

Bernstein agrees with our earlier statement that narratives arise from something; they are moments of choosing "relevant" facts that paint a new picture. He goes beyond this, however, to point out that narratives make these "facts" "meaningful" by directing them toward "future events." That is, purpose infuses the story, shaping its content and form. This is a *genuinely creative moment.* A story is "constructed" in order to make sense of lived experience. This making is artistic (as in the Greek term *poièsis*). Any storyteller, therefore, is an artist.

The "successful" story, then, takes up "facts" in order to further the imaginative elements of the story's purpose. Through this descriptive/creative interplay, the individual imagines herself situated within a community as she brings forth her unique story as a byproduct of the communities in which she participates. The stories we tell place us into community with others. This storytelling as (self-) description and (self-) creation, in turn, makes us accountable to others in their own accounts, evaluations, actions, and so forth.

But we must also consider who is creating the story. John Hardwig correctly points out that storytelling cuts both ways, for we not only tell stories about ourselves but others as well (Hardwig 1997). "Biography," then, and not just "autobiography," raises very important questions concerning who is telling the story and what that person's own position, powers, and motives are. For example, in the medical setting, is it the patient or physician who is telling the story? And is the story being told about the patient? medicine? the physician? or what? How does the story differ when the patient tells a story about herself and when the physician tells a story about the patient?

Arthur Frank illustrates the problem of "authorship" through his own personal illness experience:

> I began to realize that . . . any sense that was to be made of my experience was going to have to come from me. They [the physicians] were telling the story of my illness, but this story was not my experience, and if I was not to lose the experience that was mine, and lose part of myself with it, I needed to tell my own story. (Frank 1997, 32)

Personal stories, for Frank, empower the teller, taking back experience that might otherwise be lost. However, it is clear that we must not only tell our stories but tell stories about one another. Physicians *must* "retell" the story of the patient in the context of the physician's own practices. And yet, "the ill person should realize that physicians, whatever their intentions, have a different job description and take their stories from different communities" (Frank 1997, 45).

Frank's comments imply and caution that narratives are creative in other ways as well. The hearer, reader, or interpreter of the story is also part of this creative process. Communication that occurs between and among individuals takes both careful crafting, on the one hand, and sensitive, generous, imaginative interpretation, on the other. Herein lies one of the great strengths and weaknesses of a narrative approach, for while stories paint pictures that create novel insight, they are subject to interpretation and investigation from all members of the community for and in which they are told. To become a good interpreter, however, can take hard work to mold "literarily" sensitive habits. This is no offhand moral point, for the generous interpreter is herself *responsible* for the retelling of the story (if only to herself).

In medical encounters, these narrative insights, then, require that both physicians and patients not only become good "writers" but "readers." They must become interpreters who filter stories through the ongoing cultural/personal narrative of the reader in order to make them fit within the reader's own framework. Both physicians and patients must work on their skills of literary interpretation and their abilities to fit stories together, however, *without doing great violence to the accounts given by others*. This is no simple skill easily cultivated. It takes practice to create such intelligent habits.

Of course, as Tristram Engelhardt correctly points out, there is an asymmetry in the healing relationship that, if gone unrecognized, may stifle positive narrative exchange:

> Patients, when they come to see a health care professional, are in unfamiliar territory. They enter a terrain of issues that has been carefully defined through the long history of the health care professions. A patient is unlikely to present[14] for care with as well-analyzed and considered judgments as those possessed by health care professionals. Professionals have a community of colleagues to reinforce their views and to sustain them in their recommendations. In addition, the interchange of health care professional and patient is defined by the language of health care. Pains, disabilities, and even fears are translated into the special jargon of the health care professions. (Engelhardt 1986, 256)

To be a patient, as Richard Zaner has noted, is to be in a compromised position of *having* to trust the physician, while to be a physician is to have the history, technology, and language of the institution of medicine supporting your position of power (cf. Zaner 1988). Thus, power within the institution of medicine in which patients find themselves when at their most compromised is in the hands of their caregivers, and the danger of losing their stories in the face of this asymmetrical medical encounter, as Frank pointed out, is ever present.

Therefore, the physician is charged with the greater moral burden in many instances, having to work to provide a space for the patient's story in the patient's own language. The physician must also work to develop a story of medicine and of the particular encounter in which the patient can find herself. Meanwhile, the patient should strive to develop the medical story as her story—make it account for her life, and include her desires and interests.

But for the patient to find that voice, it often takes a physician who is sensitive both to people and to narrative and not simply a physician who is technically competent. In turn, this implies that physicians must be well trained not only in the biomedical sciences, but in human, social affairs. I take it that this is what Edmund Pellegrino has in mind at the end of his article "The Anatomy of a Clinical Judgment" when he calls for humanities education in medical school:

> If medicine is a science, and art . . . medical students will need a more explicit education in the non-scientific components of clinical judgment. . . . The liberal arts, and the humanities . . . need vigorous refurbishment in medical education where it will become more obvious to the student that he *needs* the liberal attitude of mind to function fully as a physician. (Pellegrino 1979, 191–92)

Still further, however, my discussion implies that physicians and patients both must become moral philosophers (in James's sense) and moral artists (in Fesmire's and Dewey's sense). They must work through moral imagination to include as many interests as possible of those involved or related to the encounter. No simple, principled approach will do, nor will straightforward technical competence. We must be artists, creatively invoking technology and scientific knowledge in the stories of people—that is, selves in community and enculturated. We must account for their interest as related in their stories in order to use technical abilities in successful ways; as Dewey says,

> What is relied upon is personal contact and communication; while personal attitudes, going deeper than the mere asking of questions, are needed in order to establish the confidence which is a condition for the patient's telling the story of his past. . . . [O]rganic modification is there—it is indispensable. . . . But this is not enough. The physical fact has to be taken up into the context of personal relations between human being and human being before it becomes a fact of the living present. (LW13, 334)

It is the patient's "telling the story" that must be taken into account by the physician. This accounting must then be sensitive to "personal relations between human being and human being" in order to fashion a truly moral solution. In this way, the physician is an artist whenever she moves away from general principles and instead is attentive to the individual patient and that person's story. Whenever the physician works to read the story of the patient as a socially situated human being in the writing of the medical encounter, there the physician is artistic. Again, from Dewey,

> Just in the degree in which a physician is an artist in his work he uses his science, no matter how extensive and accurate, to furnish him with tools of inquiry into the individual case, and with methods of forecasting a method of dealing with it. Just in the degree in which, no matter how great his learning, he subordinates the individual case to some classification of diseases and some generic rule of treatment, he sinks to the level of the routine mechanic. His intelligence and his action become rigid, dogmatic, instead of free and flexible. (MW12, 176)

The dogmatic physician loses sight of narrative and moral imagination, and replaces this with "routine mechanics." However, there is an alternative. The physician and patient can both attend to the details of human living as expressed through the stories they tell. This requires moral imagination. Here we do not simply have biomedical manipulation, but true medical and moral artistry.

This discussion of narrative, then, speaks to issues at the very heart of an account of moral rationality—one that rejects the "standard account of moral rationality" that is characterized by the use of rules and principles.[15] This is precisely our earlier account of moral artistry from the first chapter; it is an account that recognizes the function of creative intelligence through dramatic rehearsal and imagination, which helps to craft truly moral relationships. As Frank has put it quite strongly, "Our moral practices are our stories—we tell our stories—we make them public and hold ourselves accountable to them—in our moral practices" (Frank 1997, 39).

PERSONAL SIGNIFICANCE IN COMMUNITY[16]

After criticizing biomedical ethics principles generally, and the principle of autonomy in particular, I have enlisted the help of pragmatist philosophers and narratives—that is, life stories—to put forth my positive account of selves as social products. We are individuals always-already in community with others, and these social relationships shape the very selves we are. But one common critique of this viewpoint is that in its so-called communitarian leanings, it runs the risk of subordinating individual interests to those of the community.[17]

I have just argued, however, that a sensitivity to understanding personal stories of and by individuals gives credit to both their unique individuality as well as to the community and culture in which that individuality arises. In this section, I shall take this further by arguing, in the words of Bernstein, that stories help "bring about dramatic, i.e. meaningful, changes. A change is meaningful in relation to past and future events." We bring meaning to our lives through the stories we *enact*, and in particular, the descriptive/creative interplay in stories gives them meaning. That is, the very *meanings* of our life stories are to be found in our individual *and* communal—or better yet, individually communal—experiences coupled with the imaginative projections we extrapolate from those experiences. We are "meaning" seekers. Through our daily activities and life plans, we work to give purpose to our existences. And this is no less true (and maybe even more importantly noted) for the lives of patients who find themselves in the midst of their personal experiences of illness.

Following James, I believe that we create meaning in our own lives every time we couple some personally and intelligently conceived goal or ideal with the courage and labor necessary to achieve it. A life gains significance through intelligence and fortitude. James explains,

> The significance of life . . . is . . . the offspring of a marriage of two different parents, either of whom alone are barren. The ideals taken by themselves give no reality, the virtues by themselves no novelty. . . . [T]he thing of deepest—or at any rate, of comparatively deepest—significance in life does seem to be its character of *progress,* or that strange union of reality with ideal novelty which it continues from one moment to another to present. (James [1899b] 1977, 657)[18]

An individual progresses in life whenever she is able to develop an end and deploy means to attain it within her lived experience. For example, a student's pursuit of a medical degree gives meaning to her life as she progresses through medical school in order to become a physician. The activity is meaningful precisely for the reason that it entails a personal ideal (becoming a physician) and the wherewithal to achieve the ideal (the strength of character to succeed at the four-year grind through medical school).

Of course, simpler, less time-consuming, nonprofessional ideals and labors (such as desiring to eat and then preparing a meal) are in their own ways instances of meaningful progress, for it is our everyday labors that develop the character of our grander schemes, while grander schemes help to shape the development of everyday pursuits. Our daily ideals often become part of the means to yet further ideals, and still are themselves ends to be enjoyed without recourse to their function in our higher goals. Again, medical school, for example, takes many individual efforts that come together to produce the final degree, and each activity— for example, learning the basic medical sciences as well as taking anatomy lab, clinical skills training, and bioethics classes—can be satisfying and enjoyable in its own right, and quite independent of the connections to the whole.

Every person at any stage of life can have ideals. James further claims, "[T]here is nothing absolutely ideal: ideals are relative to the lives that entertain them" (James [1899a] 1977, 656). Meaning in life is highly individualized. For James, there simply is no overarching meaning to life; there are only the particular instances of meaning created by a particular person in the full context of that in-dividual's life. And this process of meaning begins when the "novelty" of an "in-tellectually conceived" goal takes hold of the attention and calls forth available habits and abilities into action. James states explicitly that ideals worthy of pur-suit must be both "intellectually conceived" and have "novelty at least for him whom the ideal grasps." That is, ideals must reside in reflective consciousness and take hold of individuals uniquely.

"Novelty" denotes this quality of uniqueness exemplified by possible ends as they are experienced by an individual. Ideals that "grasp" an individual take hold of the individual's attention and move her to action. The idealizer finds in the ideal the possibility for unique expression of her talents. And even though some goals may seem mundane to others, for the person who is "grasped," a sense of engagement is felt where an individual's abilities and creativity are called forth. "Sodden routine is incompatible with ideality, although *what is sodden routine for one person may be ideal novelty for another*" (James [1899b] 1977, 656 [em-phasis mine]). The ideal itself is further shaped by a person's individualized ap-proach to it. Take the example of flying. Some individuals (my father-in-law, to name one) find a joy, a "freedom," a "rush" in being up in the sky in control of an airplane. For you or me, there may be no great novelty in flight school, ground checks, aerobatics, and so forth, but it is obviously the case that individuals like Chuck Yeager, as well as my father-in-law and other hobbyists, find the act of controlled soaring through clouds an outlet for their individual and unique talents. Furthermore, there can be moments of historic novelty when particular individu-als idealize for an entire epoch (becoming "ideals" themselves)—for example, no one flies like the late, great Charles Lindbergh or Amelia Earhart. More common, however, are the daily engagements by any one of us as we pursue our desirable ends—for example, my father-in-law's love for flight.

"Intellectually conceived," on the other hand, takes us beyond mere novelty; it signifies the need, *before pursuit*, for reflection upon our ends in light of means available. Intelligent ideals are those that arise from the fusion of the descrip-tive/creative function of an acceptable, coherent story; they "fit" within the means available and other ends that have been put forth in the situation. As we have noted in chapter 1 about the continuum between means and ends, James points out that reflection takes mere valu*ed* objects—also known as descriptive "facts"—and makes them valu*able*—that is, creatively conceived goals. Intelligently conceived ideals are not simply something desir*ed* as ends in themselves, but are discovered to be desir*able* upon investigation of costs and consequences. They are, therefore, *worthy* of our desire. This use of intelligence is what situates personal goals in the complex of the communal environment in which the goals arise and are to be played out. In other words, this process is an acknowledgment that it is the narra-tive, *socially* situated self that makes ideals meaningful.

For example, a physician may wish to order a battery of tests, but the desire alone is not enough to make it worthy of pursuit. The physician must investigate the concerns raised by the expressed symptoms, the interests of the patient and others affected by the decision, economic factors, availability, time constraints, and so on. Only after having followed out this inquiry can the physician move from a mere "whimsical" ideal to something that is determined to be either valuable or not. "Whimsical" desires without reflection, no matter how much they capture the attention, rarely come to fruition and make for the possibility of unforeseen conflict down the line should we try to fulfill them. Intelligence helps us sort through (or better yet, intelligence is the sorting through of) various ends-in-view and the means available to achieve them in order to determine those "worth the effort."

These requirements of "novelty" and "intelligence" imply that ideals do not reside beyond experience as formal or absolute ends. They are created within and by our daily lives; that is, they arise out of our ongoing stories as well as the stories of those with whom we come in contact. As both intellectually conceived and novel, ideals must touch us and come to fruition in our experiences employing means available *and* accounting for others' ends as well. Admittedly, "[T]aken nakedly, abstractly, and immediately, you see that mere ideals are the cheapest things in life. Everybody has them in some shape or other, personal or general, sound or mistaken, low or high" (James [1899b] 1977, 657). However, significance in life cannot stop with "cheap" ideals. As James insists, the means employed are of equal importance to the ends, and the means also arise out of our experiences, our life stories. An ideal must be not only immediately and abstractly desired but also wedded to the discipline and courage needed to pursue it. If personal ends are to become fulfilled (within experience), we must back our "ideal visions with what the laborers have, the sterner stuff of . . . virtue; we must multiply [the ideals'] sentimental surface by the dimension of the active will, if we are to have *depth*, if we are to have anything cubical and solid in the way of character" (James [1899b] 1977, 657). Again, we see that a continuum of means and ends exists such that the means employed give otherwise empty, flighty ideals content and character. Significance, then, comes from this active striving to actualize our personal goals.

To restate, "significance" develops from a fusion of personal, particular ideals with courage, strength, and intelligence—that is, the virtues that drive people to embody these ideals in their daily lives. James's term for this is "progress," and progress incorporates the intellectual ability to create goals and the fortitude to fulfill them, regardless of our current location on the timeline between birth and death. Also, whereas fortitude and strength are sometimes difficult to muster, ideals arise everywhere; they are part and parcel of our daily lives; they are "the cheapest things in life."[19]

Meaningful living, then, is highly individualized, but always with communal content. Ideals themselves arise from our experiences in and of our communities and environments. And our intellectual support and courageous activities in pursuit of our ideals both take into account and come home to rest in this actual lived experience. In this way, it should be clear that meaning is not merely "voluntary"

and "subjective." As I have argued throughout my account of narrative significance, the stories we tell, and the meanings they convey, arise from and feed back
into the community. They are open for approval, disapproval, consternation, dis-
agreement, reconstruction, and/or acceptance by ourselves and others. In this
way, they are, or become, as "objective" as can be. Also, as open for social investigation and evaluation, the meanings of our narratives are themselves part of
the moral fabric of experience.

I have not here argued for the validity of the pragmatist position on narrative
selves and community so much as I have attempted to elucidate it. Clearly, the
implications of the pragmatist position are far-reaching for moral theory and
practice. For our purposes, this account contrasts with and supplants the current
account of moral rationality in bioethics with its use of principles and emphasis
on autonomy. Implications of my position for a variety of bioethics issues will be
taken up in the following chapter, and the issues raised in this chapter introduce
and ground the work of that which follows.

NOTES

1. We could say that children cry when they are "uncomfortable," but the *cognitive*
character that even this minimal description implies is simply not there for most infants
most of the time. Children cry, and they *know* not why, but they do in fact *have* experiences that result in "discomfort" and crying.
2. Parts of this section are revised from Hester 1998.
3. Heather Keith, in an unpublished paper (Keith 1997) on Mead's concept of "self,"
correctly points out that community involves not just individuals but the environment in
which they live. Keith explains, "The experience of being human, philosophical and biological, depends on a variety of 'ecological' relationships," and she calls this "life in a social ecology." This "ecological" aspect of community, though not explicitly discussed in
its relationship to the "natural" environment within this book, resides in the background of
any discussion of "community" contained herein.
4. For Buchler's take on community, see chapter 2, "Communication," in Buchler
(1979, 29–57).
5. The recognition of "sameness-in-difference" with emphasis on "difference" is quite
important, for it requires of us that we take difference seriously when fashioning communities. Gender, ethnicity, sexuality, and other cultural aspects of individuals must be
understood and taken into account in our moral deliberations. The insights of feminism,
ethnic/cultural sociology, and "queer" studies are but a few of the places we need to look
in order to develop better this "normative" community about which I am writing.
6. Robert Westbrook has argued that Dewey's conception of "community" appears
overly idealistic, thus failing on Dewey's own pragmatic grounds. But as Michael Eldridge
has, in turn, pointed out, Dewey's "faith" in democratic community is never *overly* ideal
but rather both (1) practically (findable in lived experience) and (2) fallibly (open to error
and adjustment) ideal. Eldridge argues that, first, both this "sharing of activities" does

happen in lived experience and the awareness and adjustments that occur because of that awareness is constitutive of the experience of community. In a simple example, marriage (in the narrowest sense) as a community of two individuals often loses its "feeling"—that is, the "experience"—of community when important conflicts arise dividing the partners; for example, when the goals of each are not shared by the other, such as desire to live in one place rather than another, or the pursuit of one profession over another. During these occasions, we may not say that the community dissolves completely (though at times it may) but certainly the experience of community does. Second, Dewey never holds this notion of community up as the absolute end; instead, he asks us to experiment with it and toss out his hypothesis if it leads to error. Further, Eldridge argues that Dewey's "ideal" of community has never been adequately attempted and implemented. Thus, we cannot say whether or not his conception works. Cf. Eldridge 1996.

7. Cf. Mead [1934] 1962, 154. Here, Mead uses the example of a baseball team in order to illustrate his notion of the "generalized other" that acts as a normative account of community where individual action is regulated by the imaginative take on what "generalized other"—that is, the other taken not as a specific person, but as a community—will do.

8. Note how the team and the management both had to adjust after the trades of ace pitcher Randy Johnson (1999) and star center fielder Ken Griffey Jr. (2000); adjustments, by the way, that resulted in a solid team that earned a spot in the American League playoffs in 2000.

9. It is important to note at this point that a social "good" itself must have a certain character to it. In particular, I take the Roycean/Deweyan position that social goods must be developed out of the interests (as diverse and conflicting as they may be) of the members of the social group and must be, what we might call, "inclusive." That is, goals of a community must be of such a character that they do not intrinsically oppose or deny the worth of alternative communities' ends unless those ends are themselves exclusive, violent, or stifling of the possibilities for a deeply enriching experience both for their members and, particularly, nonmembers—for example, a band of robber barons or the Nazi party. Josiah Royce sees this as constitutive of true "loyalty," and Dewey takes this to be the nature of a true democracy. See Royce 1995, particularly lecture 3, "Loyalty to Loyalty," 48–69; and Dewey, LW2, 235–72, particularly chapter 5, "The Search for the Great Community," 325–50. Since this discussion pertains to the health care community and its end of "health," let me say up front that I see no *intrinsically* exclusive character to "health," and so find no need to defend the mere possibility that the health care community can become an instance of an "ideal" community like I propose.

10. I might be considered negligent if I did not point out that Gilligan's work has been attacked over the years from many sides; particularly, of late, it has undergone charges of being "scientifically invalid" from Christina Hoff Sommers (2000). In my all-to-brief look at these charges, I do not find them persuasive.

11. It is also important to make clear that I am using narratives and stories in a functional, not foundational way. That is, I am not arguing that narratives are *the* mode in which selves come to be or that they are the *basis* of morality (cf. Chambers 1999). I am, however, arguing that understanding the functionality of narratives can *help* us gain perspective on how selves come to be and can be *useful* (i.e., instrumental) in working through moral dilemmas. Hilde Nelson has argued that the use of narrative in ethics can be segregated into five categories: reading stories, telling stories, comparing stories, literary analysis of stories, and invoking stories (Nelson 1997, x–xii). For me, all of the above

can be helpful to understand better the ethical aspects of experience. In what follows, however, I concentrate on the first three categories. For excellent discussions of several perspectives on the use of narratives in bioethics, see the essays in Nelson 1997.

12. Surely there can be times of so-called "discontinuity" where "epiphany," or "revelation," or "radical transformation" in, through, or of narratives occurs. But even these moments do not begin from a formless void; instead they are reworkings of elements that already exist in experience with elements new to the situation.

13. I see no easy way of retaining this term, even through reconstruction, without the risk of backsliding to this Enlightenment position.

14. The term "present" here seems a quite unfortunate use of medical language in that it is clearly passive and objectifying in tone. It is particularly surprising that someone of Engelhardt's sensitivities has been seduced by medical language in this way.

15. I am deliberately using the phrase used by Burrell and Hauerwas to describe utilitarian and deontological ethics since they argue explicitly that narrative can offer an alternative account of moral rationality to this "standard" (Burrell and Hauerwas 1979, 159–77).

16. The section is highly revised from a portion of an earlier article (Hester 1999).

17. For a discussion and critique of communitarianism and its nemesis, liberalism, from a pragmatist's standpoint, see Talisse 2000.

18. James does qualify this idea of "significance" employed here with the phrase "for communicable and publicly recognizable purposes." I believe this qualification is made to contrast with remarks he makes elsewhere in such works as *Varieties of Religious Experience* where he admits to the possibility of a kind of mystical "private" significance in an individual's life. Cf. James [1902] 1958, 292–328, lectures 16 and 17, "Mysticism." In particular, James's qualifier seems to contrast specifically with his use of the term "mystical states of consciousness" in *Varieties* where James begins his definition of this term with the idea that the mystical is "ineffable," "transient," and "passive"—three terms not readily applicable to socially recognizable meaning in life. Since my discussion is concerned with lived, social experience, James's qualifier becomes unnecessarily redundant.

19. It should be noted that we would be wise to cultivate the ability, particularly as we become elderly and our means reduce in number and potency, to find meaning more and more in those activities that youth affords us the luxury of ignoring. Rather than shaping meaning through the development of long-term goals and activities, as we age and move closer to dying (though I do not wish to restrict this only to the elderly), we should attempt to develop significance out of the more immediate pleasures and basic activities of life. As we find our abilities change, our goals must also. The less stamina and strength we demonstrate, wisdom tells us, the more immediate our ends should become. The sounds of the day, the taste of the food, the movements of the body, all can be sources of meaning. If sight begins to degenerate, simply hearing the song of a bird can be an activity both idealized and appreciated. When a hot day diminishes energy, the sensation of flavorful ice cream flowing coolly down the throat can reinvigorate. As muscles begin to weaken, the swinging of the legs and arms in everyday walking can prove defiant against the aging process. In this way, we can retain meaning throughout life by pursuing ends appropriate to our means.

Chapter 5

Community As Healing

INTRODUCTION

I have just argued above, among other things, one important point—namely, our lives are not ours alone. In order to be selves, we must first be with others. As we will see even more strikingly in this chapter, throughout our lives, our actions affect and are affected by others. Our relationships make us and mold us, and in turn, we help shape the communities around us with our novel acts of meaning as we write the stories of our lives. As moral artists we strive to weave our narratives with others in order to fashion successful encounters. The implications of these insights for physician and patient are the focus of this chapter. In particular, if insular individuality, and, thereby, the principle of autonomy, has been shown to be, at best, an incomplete account; if meaningful acts by individuals implicate others in morally important ways; and if self and community are fundamentally inextricable in lived experience, then the standard principle-based account of moral interactions between health care professionals and patients must go.

I, therefore, offer my alternative to the traditional bioethical theories. It is an account based in the pragmatic tradition of William James, John Dewey, and George Herbert Mead. It recognizes the self as social product to the extent that healthy living for any self means living an integrated life in community with others. As such, medical encounters are well described as attempts to place, when possible, disconnected patients back into their larger community contexts, but not only this; for medical encounters, in order to be most effective, must recognize the all-important continuum between ends and means. Thus, if community participation is the end of the encounter, it should also be implicated in the means to that end. Patient participation within a community of healing is, therefore, essential to a "healing" encounter. These kinds of encounters treat patients as members of the health care community, a community that, ideally, mirrors the form and function of the larger community in which it resides.[1] This "community" emphasis

67

is best accomplished through the promotion of patient agency—namely, allowing the patient to act meaningfully—within the medical encounter itself. That is, this is best accomplished, not by way of championing the principle of autonomy through informed consent (which is fine as far as it goes), but through *participation* in "community as healing."

A BREAK WITH "EVERYDAY" EXPERIENCE

After an automobile accident in January of 1986, a sixty-five-year-old, active artist (a painter called Mr. I.) was left without an ability to see color. Noted author and neurologist Oliver Sacks recounted the immediate aftermath:

> The weeks that followed were very difficult. "You might think," Mr. I. said, "loss of color vision, what's the big deal? Some of my friends said this, my wife sometimes thought this, but to me, at least, it was awful, disgusting." He *knew* the colors of everything, with an extraordinary exactness. . . . He *knew* all the colors in his favorite paintings, but could no longer see them, either when he looked or in his mind's eye. . . . Mr. I. could hardly bear the changed appearances of people ("like animated grey statues") any more than he could bear his own appearance in the mirror: he shunned social intercourse and found sexual intercourse impossible. He saw people's flesh, his wife's flesh, his own flesh, as an abhorrent grey; "flesh-colored" now appeared "rat-colored" to him. . . . The "wrongness" of everything was disturbing, even disgusting, and applied to every circumstance of daily life. He found foods disgusting due to their greyish, dead appearance and had to close his eyes to eat. (Sacks 1995, 6–7)

As Sacks shows in this passage, bodily injury and medical disease affect persons at a social/cultural level for the obvious reason that disease and injury imply social disruption—that is, they imply illness or debilitation. At the level of cultural interaction and daily living, injury and disease manifest themselves as disruptions—disruptions of *social* vitality. An *experience* of disjunction occurs within the social integrity of the individual. That is, the biological phenomenon of disease or injury creates social disjunctions in and around the individual. As Richard Zaner points out, "Any sort of affliction, trivial or grievous, effectively breaks into the usual textures of daily life with its taken-for-granted network of concerns, interests, preoccupations, activities, and involvements" (Zaner 1988, 53). When biological disturbances within the body manifest themselves in human experience, the result is a felt disconnection from the "taken-for-granted" (or "everyday") quality of our experiences. The habits we so often rely upon, fail us. Color blindness changes fresh fruit into inedible decaying masses, broken bones force us to walk or grasp differently, the flu reduces our stamina and minimizes our ability to participate in activities, and cancer is a catalyst for feelings of mortality. These afflictions cost us time and money, and they demand concentrated efforts in order to be overcome.

Whereas Zaner shows illness to be an experienced break with "everydayness," the converse holds as well. That is, all situations that are experienced as a "break" are what John J. McDermott calls "pathological."

[A]ny situation which cripples or enervates the human organism, however unusual or vague its roots, is a pathological condition. The task of medicine conceived as a social science (which is not exclusive of medicine as a natural science) is to build into its diagnostic procedures a sensitivity to this dimension of contemporary human experience. (McDermott 1976, 170)

Discontinuities in life can lead to "crippling" or "enervating" experiences; they are diseaselike in the way we are moved or stifled in our movements to respond to them. Any experience, whether initially recognized or conceived as either biochemical or medical, is "pathological" to the degree that it diminishes vigor and vitality. McDermott's point, then, is that so long as a person resides in a situation that demoralizes and disrupts the usual flows of life, that individual is in the midst of a "pathological" experience. Thus, events experienced as stifling or frustrating to human living should be taken seriously by medicine in its practice as a "social" science of human interactions. The purview of medicine, then, is greatly extended from the narrow realm of biology to the greater scope of social intercourse, implying an infinite plurality of medical situations.

Because an illness experience is different for each ailment and each patient, medical encounters fall along a continuum. This continuum ranges from relatively less problematic cases to the more complex, from those situations of injury or illness that have fairly "straightforward" solutions and threaten the integrity of the self very little—for example, a cut on the leg that is stitched up and heals, a broken arm that mends without complications—to debilitating chronic or terminal illness that can call into question virtually every aspect and relationship of living—such as end-stage renal failure or widely metastasized lung cancer.

In so-called "simpler" cases, patients and physicians alike might be perfectly willing to deal almost exclusively with the ailment and virtually ignore further concerns of the patient's life. A person who cuts her nondominant hand while slicing the morning bagel can often do enough damage to merit a drive to the emergency room or local walk-in "urgent care" facility. However, the encounter that ensues is often unproblematic medically, socially, and personally. Aside from a possible long wait (which is not wholly unimportant), for many people a few simple words, a quick investigation, and some stitches do the trick; relatively little else is required by either party. One reason for this is that the cut, though annoying, is rarely experienced as detrimental to active functioning in the world. Psychological distancing is relatively easy, and injuries of this sort are rarely felt to inhibit or disturb the patient's sense of self. It may seem crass, but in cases like these, the medical encounter is not wholly unlike daily encounters with engineers, mechanics, or other knowledgeable service professionals. Bodily injury or illness, in these situations, is often experienced as "other" to self.

As we move along the continuum to more and more complex cases, however, a deeper appreciation of the complete life of the patient—that is, interests, values, obligations, relationships, and so on—becomes necessary. Chronic kidney disease infuses itself into the very texture of life. Not only do patients have to undergo hemodialysis, but fatigue, pain, and stress accompany virtually all activity. The patient's life habits are not only taxed, they are called into question, changed completely, or left behind entirely. In these cases, selves are intimately involved and dissolved, repaired and compared. For medicine to help these patients effectively, relationships must be forged and strengthened, relationships must make room for and promote patients' narratives and participations.

Of course, my brief account of the continuum simplifies a highly complex issue, for each patient will react differently to an ailment (just as any particular encounter with an engineer or mechanic may be more or less disruptive to our daily lives). For example, regardless of where you or I might place an illness like influenza along the continuum, any particular patient might experience it as anywhere from a simple nuisance to a basic hindrance to a severe threat. Thus, we cannot categorize medical encounters a priori according to aliments and how they will be experienced; that is, we cannot say ahead of time what any particular medical encounter might entail, especially with regard to the experiences of ailments by the patient. But what we can say is that the more complex and threatening the experience for the patient, the more it tears at the fabric of that person's life. And conversely, *the more an ailment tears at the fabric of our relationships, the more severely it is experienced.*

Returning, then, to Zaner's insight (portrayed by Sacks's artist), we find that in cases of illness, and particularly in more severe and/or chronic cases, our relationships to others are reconceived. We experience others—even those intimately related to us—as changed or distant, we find ourselves demanding extra help from friends and family, we miss work, we require treatment from health care professionals, and we reevaluate future aspirations and the character of our relationships. Disease (dis-ease) or injury arrests our abilities to function within our accustomed habits. It jars us in our relationship to self and others and disturbs our ongoing life stories. Thus, "pathologies" (in McDermott's words) from an experiential perspective tear at our social life—that is, at our lived experiences of social integrity and vitality. They call into question the very ability to fulfill obligations as well as reach desired ends. Disease or injury creates a break between the individual and the community that compromises the individual's status within the community and compromises the integrity of the self as a "product" of social interaction (recall the argument of the previous chapter).

The problem encountered in the experience of medical disease or injury is that the relationships that make up an individual's experience of community are, if not severed, compromised. Our "everyday" activities are called into question since our abilities to fulfill our obligations and to achieve many of our ends are diminished through the weakening of our bodies. Exemplified by Sacks's artist, Zaner's point about illness and the "textures" of life is that even in small ways, being stricken with some illness means that our taken-for-granted activities are called into question and our most intimate relationships must be adjusted in order to fulfill our roles in society. Returning to our earlier example, the patient with end-stage renal failure is placed on dialysis and the United Network for Organ Sharing (UNOS) waiting list for an organ transplant.[2] The time taken each week to perform dialysis and the time spent waiting for an organ emphasize the felt sense of disintegration with the environment and community that the patient goes through. Particularly, a patient whose self is thrust into question by an ailment realizes, "I am not healthy. I cannot perform without medical intervention. People treat me differently. My ability to carry out my obligations to family, friends, job, and so on, are compromised. I will either lose everything or reinvent my*self*."

Dewey himself points to this phenomenon when he says, "What are the resulting pathological phenomena but evidences that the self loses its integrity *within itself* when it loses integration with the medium [both somatic and social] in which it lives?" (LW13, 328–29). Self and environment are connected in healthy living. Disease, illness, and injury separate the patient from community by disrupting the individual's social life plan—narrative—and the social connections that make up that person's life.

> The person who is ill not merely suffers pain but is rendered unfit to meet his ordinary social responsibilities; he is incapacitated for service to those about him, some of whom may be directly dependent upon him. Moreover, his removal from the sphere of social relations does not merely leave a blank where he was; it involves a wrench upon the sympathies and affections of others. (LW2, 99)

We become afflicted; our lives are changed, and with those changes, others, too, are affected. As we have noted throughout, clearly our lives are not atomic and insular. Our actions affect and are affected by others. Illness itself causes us to be displaced from our usual patterns within our spheres of influence. Family, friends, and coworkers are asked to "make up the difference" and fill the social void left by our absences.

LIVING *HEALTHILY*

In light of what we have just said about disease and illness, it should be evident that healing should be concerned with restoring the individual to a state of vital functioning, and vital functioning entails communal participation.

> To cure disease and prevent death is to promote the fundamental conditions of social welfare; is to secure the conditions requisite to an effective performance of all social activities; is to preserve human affections from the frightful waste and drain occasioned by the needless suffering and death of others with whom one is bound up. (LW2, 99)

According to this account, health care is about "preserving human affections"—
that is, providing patients with the means to retain or restore their relationships to
others within the community.

However, as seen in our discussion of Pellegrino in chapter 1, good clinical
medicine, far from the generalities of "pure science," is always concerned with
the particular ends of actual patients. In this light, Dewey reminds us that the end
of any medical encounter, though concerned with community, must be taken individually. "How to live healthily . . . is a matter which differs with every person.
It varies with his past experience, his opportunities, his temperamental and acquired weaknesses and abilities" (MW12, 175). So as we see in the Sacks story
above, Mr. I.'s affliction may seem trivial to others—namely, his wife and
friends—but to him nothing could have been more detrimental to his personal
pursuits and the abilities he had cultivated over a lifetime. His experience of the
world was fundamentally shaped by the colors he saw and the meaning those colors provided to his life's story. In order to live healthily, he had to find a way either to recapture those color experiences or rehabituate his activities in light of
his new circumstances. Dewey captures this need to integrate actively our desires
and current situations when he explains,

> Healthy living is not something to be attained by itself apart from other ways of liv-
> ing. A man needs to be healthy *in* his life, not apart from it, and what does life mean
> except the aggregate of his pursuits and activities? . . . Surely, once more, what a man
> needs is to live healthily, and this result so affects all the activities of his life that it
> cannot be set up as a separate and independent good. (MW12, 175)

Note that Dewey avoids the use of the noun "health," preferring instead to concentrate on the adverb "healthily." Nouns denote static "things," but what Dewey
emphasizes is that we are not talking here about any static condition of human beings. As he says, "To say a man seeks health . . . is only to say that he seeks to
live healthily. . . . [This is] adverbial. [It is a] modifier of action in special cases"
(MW12, 175).[3] Health as "living healthily" emphasizes the modification of our
actions and pursuits constantly present in a healthy life. "Living healthily" is not
a static state of being; it is instead the condition of actively pursuing meaningful
goals and developing your*self* by accounting for both your ongoing story line and
the current demands of the environment.

This is exemplified in Mr. I.'s own healing process:

> Immediately after his accident, and for a year or more thereafter, Jonathan I. insisted
> that he still "knew" colors. . . . But, thereafter, he became somewhat less sure, as if
> now, unsupported by actual experience or image, his color associations had started
> to give way. . . . There was a lessening concern with what he had lost, and indeed
> with the whole subject of color, which had first so obsessed him. Indeed, he now
> spoke of being "divorced" from color. . . . At once forgetting and turning away from
> color, turning away from the chromatic orientation and habits and strategies of his

previous life, Mr. I., in the second year after his injury, found that he saw best in subdued light or twilight, and not in the full glare of day. . . . He started becoming a "night person," in his own words, and took to exploring other cities, other places, but only at night. . . . "Gradually I am becoming a night person. It's a different world: there's a lot of space—you're not hemmed in by streets, by people. . . . It's a whole new world." (Sacks 1995, 35–37)

Losing his color vision, so important to him as the painter he once was, forces Mr. I. to reorient his life habits, rewriting his life story. At first stifled by his affliction, he turns to the world of the night, actively reconstructing himself. In becoming a "night person," Mr. I. finds and creates a "whole new world"—a world in which he can once again actively pursue goals of interest to him. Further, Mr. I. begins the process of reconnecting with others in his activities by "occasionally talking with a fellow walker, occasionally going into little diners," no longer afraid of the "grey statues" (Sacks 1995, 37). These new habits, new orientations, and new interactions—that is, the activities of his new narrative self—illustrate that healthy living always makes reference to one's social/experiential conditions. Selves and their activities cannot be separated from the context of their respective environments, of interactions and exchanges. Mr. I.'s actions show that living healthily is the process of integrated lived experience (between environment, self, and community) where one actively participates in the creation of her own life story and, even if only in small ways, the activities of others.

CONTINUUM BETWEEN MEANS AND ENDS IN HEALTH CARE

We have already noted briefly in chapters 1 and 4 that means and ends can never be strictly divorced from each other. As we are reminded by Ernest Nagel, commenting on some of Dewey's insights, "The character of means employed enters constitutively into the character of ends attained" (Nagel 1986, ix). Our ends are only attainable through the means available, and the means used are chosen and take on their specific characteristics as means given the ends for which they are employed. The ends and means within health care relationships and activities are no different. Medicine, as has been previously noted, is concerned with reaching the end of health, or better yet, "living healthily."

This active process of living healthily is highly individualized, but, as we have also noted, this should not be confused with the belief that individuals are insular and atomic. Though each of us uniquely participates in the world, our very selves are shaped by the communities in which we find ourselves. And, as I have been arguing throughout this chapter, living healthily implies connection with the communities in which we regularly participate. That is, living healthily, far from achieving some state of atomic, autonomous control, is the process of interacting with others of our community and being recognized as members of relatively equal standing.

As illustrated by Sacks's artist, community seeking is one thing patients do. If a community is not provided for them during their encounters with health care professionals (and even sometimes when it is), patients will seek other avenues. James Buchanan in his book *Patient Encounters* writes about one such patient with amyotrophic lateral sclerosis (ALS).

> Stanley Derek Ackroyd, Ph.D. (in philosophy), was an extraordinary and exceptional person now reduced to an ordinary and perfectly predictable disease. . . . [In the face of ALS, Stanley] sought out the company of people who were ordinary, uninformed, and even quite unsophisticated. Formerly the thought of exchanging pleasantries with a cabdriver or a bellhop would have seemed preposterous, but now it had its charm. . . . Stanley liked these people, and they offered him both the community and the nonjudgmental acceptance he needed. (Buchanan 1989, 24–25)

Professor Ackroyd "needed" a community in order to feel at home in a world that had been radically altered. His circumstances and reactions embody an instance of the attempt to live healthily that functions in part both as an end of medicine and means to that end.

Both Mr. I. and Dr. Ackroyd exemplify a need rarely satisfied within medical encounters. Because the lives they knew had been greatly disrupted, they sought to find new avenues of agency, of participation, of belonging. Quite simply, they illustrate the need to connect with others in a community. That is, living healthily makes reference to an integrated living in community with others. Of course, given the important continuum between means and ends, within the limits of biological and technical possibility, the medical encounter itself should be an instance of the very same moral/social ideal previously discussed in chapter 4 for the community at large. In other words, *if living in community with others*—that is, living healthily—*is the end-in-view for medical encounters, it must also be implicated in the means to that end.* The extent to which health care providers interact with patients so as to include them within the community of healing and that community's story is the extent to which the end of "living healthily" is already satisfied within treatment itself. A patient who is given the opportunity and encouragement to participate as a member of the health care community— that is, encouraged both to find herself within the narrative of medicine and to create a narrative about herself that makes medicine an integral part of it—in order to reach the goal of living healthily in her larger community has *already* begun to live healthily because she begins to experience an integrated, situated living with a community. This requires the promotion of patient agency, the providing of space for expressions of patient interests and values in medical decision making, and the support for active participation by the patient in her own healing process. It means finding and promoting shared experience among all participants in the medical encounter—particularly between physicians and patients—working to adjust the many ongoing narratives to account adequately for each other.

However, unlike the examples from Sacks and Buchanan, where illness and debilitation caused Dr. Ackroyd and Mr. I. to look to people outside their everyday communities or to the relationships developed because of their ailments, I am urging members of the health care community to realize that they can and should provide a place for patients such as Dr. Ackroyd and Mr. I. as members of the health care community itself. [4] I believe health care professionals should adapt their practices in light of an understanding of the constitutive character of means and ends in order to give the opportunity for active participation by the patient. [5]

The task is daunting from several perspectives. "Medical practice has traditionally been strongly paternalistic: [that is,] Physicians have often concealed diagnoses from patients 'for their own good'" (Jonsen et al. 1986, 48). Along this line, the community of health care has often not treated the patient as a member of the community but has viewed her as an "accidental tourist." This runs directly counter to patient agency. These attitudes treat experiences of being a patient as temporary states *merely* to be "gotten over." This amounts to medical encounters being merely means and never also ends (qua satisfactions) in themselves. However, the insights gained from an acknowledgment of the continuum between means and ends is that a great loss of possible satisfactions occurs when *all* moments within the encounter are to be taken merely as means to some further satisfactory moment and never as satisfactory themselves. This was nicely illustrated earlier through James's take on significance. Means and ends intermingle and coexist in such a way that when means are found to be satisfactory as ends themselves, this helps to create further meaningful, satisfactory ends as the outcome of these means.[6]

OVERCOMING ASYMMETRY AND "HUMAN BLINDNESS" THROUGH COMMUNITY

Fundamental obstacles to developing communities in medical encounters, however, need to be noted. Physicians have long held a position of authority in society at large and in medical encounters in particular. Obviously, there are important reasons for this. Physicians have a kind of knowledge not possessed by most of their patients (which is why patients seek them out), and this fact leads to an imbalance of status and power in medical encounters. In Zaner's words, "[Patients] realize that to be sick is to be disadvantaged and compromised both by the illness and by the relationship to the doctor, who has the edge over the patient in knowledge, skills, resources, and social legitimation and authority" (Zaner 1993, 10). There is a fundamental "asymmetry" in physician–patient relationships.

[This] asymmetry of power in the helping relationship is marked by the "peculiarly vulnerable existential state" of the patient and the power of the professed healer(s). . . . From the perspective of the patient, illness or injury forces breaks with the usual flow of daily life. (Zaner 1988, 55)[7]

This "break" disables the patient in ways that force the individual to place trust in the physician, "and obliges the patient to rely on the care of other persons" (Zaner 1988, 55). Meanwhile, the physician, by way of technical ability and scientific knowledge, is empowered within and by the relationship, and though most likely a stranger to the patient, is implicitly entrusted with a responsibility to help the patient. This imbalance of power, which is prima facie constitutive of physician–patient relationships, acts as a primary obstacle to communication.

We have noted in the previous chapter the dangers raised by this asymmetry as it relates to the "authoring" of life stories. We can further see this historically where physicians have exercised their authority and power through what have come to be known as "paternalistic acts." Particularly before the 1960s, physicians routinely withheld information, performed unexplained procedures, or made unilateral medical decisions, claiming that they knew what was best for their patients. In response to this and other issues, a new "bioethical" movement culminated at the end of the 1970s in the establishment of the four basic principles of biomedical ethics of Beauchamp and Childress. Specifically, as discussed in chapter 3, the principle of autonomy was invoked as a safeguard against paternalistic acts by medical professionals and was procedurally embodied in "informed consent" documentation.

Unfortunately, the changes in bioethics of the last thirty years have not been able to eradicate all traces of paternalistic habits. As Dewey has clearly explained, habits are a function of the environment as much as they are of the organism. And in the case of paternalistic medical habits, as the environment changed with regard to ethical practice, so too did the activities. The habits themselves did not disappear completely. They simply became reconstructed in order to accommodate the prevailing attitudes embraced by the social situation. Rather than "overt" acts of paternalism, the habits have become more covert. Still, in the name of "doing the best for the patient," physicians fudge the spirit of "informed consent" in favor of following its legal letter. Habituation to reading the form, accepting the signature, and moving on is common. But even more dangerous are the half-reflective habits performed under the guise of "good medicine." It is not uncommon for physicians to tell just half the story, to explain the information only in the "best possible light," or skew the information in a particular way to get a desired result.[8]

In 1996, I spent several weeknights at a local hospital as a participant in a seminar for health professionals on end-of-life issues. Each evening consisted of reading articles, a presentation by a physician, and discussion. One night, the topic focused on the "four principles" of bioethics, where the presenter listed these on a whiteboard and proceeded to explain that they were the basis for ethical practice. Uncontroversially, the assemblage (myself and another excepted) nodded in agreement. The discussion that followed was led by one physician in particular (an internist) who claimed to accept the notion of autonomy readily, yet also knew that sometimes telling the patient everything would simply cause fright. Medical knowledge on the level that the physician controlled was simply too scary for the layperson. He went on to say that since illness is a time of difficulty and compromise for the patient, he felt it his moral duty to make many decisions for the patient and to direct the tone and tenor of the conversations, relieving the patient and the family of that stress. His term for this practice was "enlightened paternalism" since he felt he had learned the lessons of the principle of autonomy and applied them consistently to his encounters with patients. Quickly and unanimously, the medical professionals in the room agreed and supported his position with similar confessions of their own.

Clearly, situations like these are dangerous for moral interaction in medicine. This story, in particular, raises at least two questions: Why is medical knowledge too frightening for some, but does not overwhelm physicians themselves, and if it does frighten physicians, even a little, why sell patients short on their ability to handle frightening, difficult information?[9] Also, what understanding of "autonomy" is at work here such that physicians see their "enlightened" paternalistic actions as ethically acceptable without argument?[10] These questions go to the heart of medical practice, for they ask about the way physicians actually interact with their patients and the attitudes displayed by these interactions.

Medical encounters with these kinds of physicians are particular instances of what James observed concerning human experience and practice:

> We are practical beings, each of us with limited functions and duties to perform. Each is bound to feel intensely the importance of his own duties and the significance of the situations that call these forth. But this feeling is in each of us a vital secret, for sympathy with which we vainly look to others. The others are too much absorbed in their own vital secrets to take an interest in ours. Hence the stupidity and injustice of our opinions, so far as they deal with the significance of alien lives. Hence the falsity of our judgments, so far as they presume to decide in an absolute way on the value of other persons' conditions or ideals. (James [1899b] 1977, 629–30)

James speaks here of the blindness of human beings to each others' duties, interests, and values—a blindness brought on by self-absorption in our own interests and values. He warns of the problems with making "absolute" judgments concerning others given this blindness in us. If we take James seriously, then we must be careful in our attempts to decide for other people concerning situations that affect them. Our self-concerned habits lead to the easy judgment that what is best for others is merely what we judge to be best for ourselves; at which point, we simply adjudicate according to our own obligations and satisfactions rather than attempt to understand other people's desires and beliefs.

On those occasions when social, physical, and mental faculties are not enough to overcome biological forces of injury or disease, we seek the aid of professionals trained in the science of medicine. We want to become reconnected with the world we once knew—that is, the everyday experiences we so often take for granted. Our illness thwarts our attempts to move along our accustomed paths.

We turn to physicians in order to find ourselves again. But, of course, if Jamesean "blindness" is true of all of us, then it is especially worth noting in the asymmetrical relationship between physicians and patients, where communication about personal ends and development of common ends is key to a positive outcome for all concerned. In our society, physicians obtain a power and status often unquestioned and highly rewarded. Patients too often accept a stereotype of the physician as all knowing. To the extent that a physician buys into this stereotype, her blindness is sure to interfere with the process of communication. The physician will attempt during the course of the relationship to fulfill the duty of healing as it is defined by her personal and professional values, while the patient will try to return to living healthily. Without relinquishing the necessary knowledge and abilities that empower physicians in their chosen profession, a certain kind of control made possible by the asymmetrical relationship must be relinquished by physicians in order to overcome the "blindness" dangerously apparent in many medical interactions. Control and "blindness" hinder a patient's ability to participate actively in that person's own healing process.

This is not to make the oxymoronic statement that it is solely within the physician's power to empower patients. Illness experiences can make patients powerless in the encounter, and they often give themselves over too easily, allowing the physician too great a say in treatment. Physicians must provide opportunities for patients to participate, yes; but patients themselves must take the responsibility of membership within the health care community as well. Both parties must make progressive, active attempts to bridge this gap and forge communal bonds. If "our human blindness" is not overcome to some reasonable degree, if the relationship is allowed to remain asymmetrical to the extent that health care professionals are merely "consented to" by patients and not "engaged with" patients and their stories, physicians and patients may work at cross-purposes, reach for different ends based on different values, never coming together for a common goal. Living healthily for the patient simply may not be understood in the same way by the physician. Having differing desires is not in itself wrong, but in order to fulfill possibly competing desires, much intelligent work must be done.

Of course, there are those so-called "easy" cases of full recovery we mentioned earlier—for example, a broken arm that heals and "goes away." Difficult problems, however, arise when a complex situation is confronted, when the subsequent state for the current patient will involve a "compromise" in which there is a continuation of aspects from the current "unhealthy" condition that carries forth into the future—for example, the artist who becomes color-blind, the professor with ALS, the elderly woman in a nursing home, or the HIV patient with a continuing regimen of drug therapy. In these cases, living healthily is not always easy to determine, for as we saw with the professor with ALS and his newfound interest in "cabdrivers" and "bellhops," the significance of "living healthily" for the patient will most likely change during the course of the physician–patient relationship. However, it is important to note that it is a change that *arises out of an already existing* set of values, interest, and obligations—that is, an existing narrative—which must now account for new medical circumstances; it is a change *from a previously conceived and currently influential* idea of living healthily *by and for* a particular patient.

Fulfilling the desire to restore a patient to health takes competent medical judgment, but it is typically judgment *by* a physician *about* a patient. These judgments are bound to be inappropriate to the extent that physicians do not engage the patient in the healing process. That is, physicians must inquire about, communicate concerning, and include patient values and interests during the "clinical judgment" process: basically, this entails understanding medical values, reflecting upon them (accepting or changing them), and weaving them with patient values (also reflected upon) in order to come to the most satisfactory solution—a solution that ideally will satisfy all claims by the individuals and institutions involved. Clearly, this takes a physician who listens to patients, invites patients into the world of medicine, and reaches into the patient's world as well.

Medicine has long equated the "technically, scientifically competent physician" with the "good physician." However,

> we need to recover from the impression, now wide-spread, that the essential problem is solved when chemical, immunological, physiological and anatomical knowledge is sufficiently obtained. We cannot understand and employ this knowledge until it is placed integrally in the context of what human beings do to one another in the vast variety of their contacts and associations. (LW13, 336)

This is not to say that technical ability and medical/scientific knowledge are superfluous. On the contrary, technical ability and sound medical knowledge are necessary, but they are not sufficient conditions for good doctoring. To understand healthy living in the context of a particular patient, a physician must not only account for biological/physiological conditions and modifications, she must investigate these conditions as they play themselves out in a particular patient's experience.

The physician, then, must work to understand the patient's past, her reflections, and the account of her story. The patient as a narrative self within not only a biological but cultural nexus must be explored, comprehended, and allowed to participate in the process of healing that is itself a moment of restoration to a state of living healthily by and for the patient. Communication must occur and trust must be built. As I have quoted before,

> What is relied upon is personal contact and communication; while personal attitudes, going deeper than the mere asking of questions, are needed in order to establish the confidence which is a condition for the patient's telling the story of his past. . . . [O]rganic modification is there—it is indispensable. . . . But this is not enough. The physical fact has to be taken up into the context of personal relations between human being and human being before it becomes a fact of the living present. (LW13, 334)

Physicians must educate themselves as humanists, not simply as "pure" scientists. The ability to "read" and interpret a patient's story is indispensable to the medical encounter when reaching for its end of living healthily. This "reading" both integrates the biological and the cultural and brings the patient into the health care community by helping the patient find herself in the story of the medical encounter as related by the physician. This implies that the patient be made a participant in her own healing process rather than simply a passive entity to be diagnosed and worked on.

Further, patients must become agents of living healthily, not simply prior to and after medical intervention, but during it as well. Patients must actively pursue the goals of their own medical encounters by engaging in the healing process—namely, by telling their stories, eliciting the stories of physicians, nurses, and others, and taking responsibility for their all-important roles in the community of health care.

All these engagements, then, recognize that "living healthily" is an integrated and active process. As an end of the medical encounter, living healthily entails the means used to reach it, and these means recognize the end of living healthily as dependent upon connections between individuals and communities. Through the inclusion of individual desires and a striving for mutual satisfaction of multiple desires, medical encounters become vehicles for communal participation by both health care professionals and patients engaged in the mutual attainment of common ends in and through living healthily.

NOTES

1. Given the passive quality of a mirror, it is important to supplement this description by saying that the health care community should not only mirror the larger community, but also (like any community member), should work to challenge and change the larger community when intelligent inquiry warrants such changes.

2. The United Network for Organ Sharing is the national organ donation network that matches patients to donated organs as they become available.

3. This is a consistent Deweyan analysis of the relationship between language and experience—for example, in the context of the use of the terms "thought" and "intelligence," Dewey states in *Experience and Nature*, "'Thought,' reason, intelligence, whatever word we choose to use, is *existentially* an adjective (*or better an adverb*), not a noun. It is a disposition of activity, a quality of . . . conduct" (LW1, 126 [emphasis mine]).

4. This is not to deny the enrichment that can be gained by involvement in communities otherwise missed or ignored. Dr. Ackroyd's newfound appreciation in people he used to overlook certainly has given his life newfound dimensions. My point is simply that if the health care community had opened itself up to the possibility of including Dr. Ackroyd as a member, he would not have been left to his own devices in his time of need.

5. There are many other communities that might be discussed here, including the important and necessary development of "peer groups" of patients coming together to form strong communities among themselves. From the political arena formed around "patients'

rights" advocates to consumer enterprises like "People's Medical Society" (see Inlander et al. 1991) to therapeutic patient groups, there are numerous ways that patients can and should form bonds through shared experiences resulting in communities of patient members. However, I am focusing primarily on the fact that the medical establishment itself must work to make patients participating members within its own practices and institutions.

6. No doubt there are medical encounters where the desire to reach an end is so great and simple enough to satisfy that "getting it over with" is an acceptable attitude—that is, there are cases that fall at the "less-complex" end of the continuum—but even these encounters *can benefit* from a focus that implicates both the ends to be reached *and* the means used to reach them.

7. Zaner's discussion of "asymmetry" is indebted to both P. B. Lenrow and Edmund Pellegrino.

8. A survey taken in the late 1970s showed clearly that practices had changed since the early 1960s. Fully, there was an 86 percent increase in the number of physicians who said that their usual policy is to tell patients when they have cancer (98 percent in 1977, up from 12 percent in 1961). However, even as the authors of the study noted, "Many questions still remain. Do physicians tell patients they have 'cancer,' or are euphemisms such as 'tumor' or 'growth' still widely used, and if so what does that mean for the communication process?" (Novack et al. 1979, 74). The question still remaining to this day is not "Do physicians talk with patients?" but "What do they say and why?"

9. There are the "routine" answers to this, of course. For example, medical knowledge is frightening for the patient because it is about the patient, not the physician—it speaks to the patient's condition. Or, medicine is frightening because it is difficult to understand and takes many years to perfect. But these responses beg the question, for they avoid the hard work—namely, they point to the fact that in order for communication to occur successfully and not covertly, much effort must be made by both parties.

10. This question is more difficult to answer than the last, but clearly, the definition of "autonomy" is, at best, "consent," and, at worst, nonexistent.

Epilogue

IMPLICATIONS FOR SIGNIFICANT WORK BEYOND THE ISSUES

Permit me one last story of a medical encounter gone wrong in order to punctuate the concerns and arguments of this book. A few years ago, I was told by a woman in her sixties about a trip to her personal physician to have a lump on her mouth examined. During the course of the examination, the physician noticed another lump on her inner thigh. The physician, concerned about its cancerous potential, referred her to a surgeon for a more thorough investigation. Later, in the surgeon's office, the lump on her leg was biopsied, and the woman was sent on her way. Several weeks had passed when the woman received a call from the office manager for the surgeon saying that the woman would have to come in for a half-hour medical procedure to remove the lump. The woman promptly asked if the lump was malignant, but the office manager said that there was nothing to worry about. They had simply encountered conflicting test results, so the surgeon wanted to remove the lump as a precaution. The office manager then reiterated that this would only be a half-hour procedure and asked when the woman could be scheduled for the operation. Skeptical (at best), the woman asked to speak with the doctor, but this required a callback since he was not immediately available. A few days later, a nurse from the surgeon's office called the woman and restated what the office manager had said. Pressing further, the woman asked how long she would be off her feet. The nurse replied that it would be a minimum of a week. The woman then asked about the "maximum." Unfortunately, the nurse could not be sure of this. So, the woman asked if it could be as many as three weeks, to which the nurse said that this was quite possible. Finally, the woman then refused the procedure and ended the conversation.

Much is going on here, but several points may help us. To look at this woman, her physical characteristics give little indication of her athletic pursuits. She is in her sixties, short, round, and seemingly frail. It turns out, however, that she is an avid skier. It was December and having the procedure would risk missing her ski season. Not only did the surgeon not get this part of the woman's story, he quite possibly "misread" her interests based on her physical appearance alone. Also, to the surgeon, as was reiterated several times by both the office manager and the nurse, the procedure was a short half hour in the office, not a three- (or possibly greater) week-long ordeal. The woman's life outside his office was not his concern except in so far as his procedure successfully or unsuccessfully removed the lump (and its possible cancerous ramifications) from her life. Finally, it is interesting to note the "disappearance" of the referring physician after the referral occurred, as well as the "disappearance" of the surgeon after the biopsy.

Still, this case could be seen as a frustrating but straightforward example of a medical encounter where the patient exercised her right to refuse treatment in accordance with the information received from the medical staff. Autonomy was respected in that there was no interference with the patient's self-determined choice once information was transmitted. Of course, it could be argued that not enough information was given to provide for truly "informed consent," but this analysis does not capture the felt sense of dissatisfaction expressed by the woman afterward. Quite simply, she was never made a member of the community. Her presence in the medical setting was treated as accidental. Her time outside the office was of no concern to the physician; it was simply a half-hour procedure. Her story was never heard since it could not be told. Her desires and pursuits were never investigated, so no solution could ever be meaningful for both parties. Further, the very fabric of the encounter left no room for her to tell her story. Her personal physician left the scene as soon as she was referred to the surgeon, and the surgeon never made room for her to express her interests to him.

If the patient is included within the health care community, if the physician takes the time to hear her story, if he himself tells a story that makes her a participant in the healing process, if the patient can view this encounter as part of her life and not an impediment to it, if it can be made meaningful for both parties, then the interactions change radically. In this way, storytelling/story-enacting integrates the medical encounter into the patient's life. The medical encounter thereby becomes an integral aspect of the patient's continuing life story. Maybe what could happen here is that a particular space and time be set aside in order to exchange narratives, maybe information could be more clearly exchanged in a mutually agreeable language, maybe several alternatives could be explored, maybe the physician and patient could work together to find a suitable solution that satisfies the interests of both, and maybe common ends could be developed and achieved.

There is a great deal of work to be done in medicine and bioethics. This book itself will not be complete until it can bear fruit beyond its own arguments and examples. Important issues in medicine: end-of-life care, reproductive technologies, organ procurement and allocation, fetal tissue research, cloning, genetic testing and engineering, as well as medical futility and care for severely impaired infants are but a few areas that need further inquiry.[1] The work left not only in my future, but also for the future of bioethics itself, is massive and inexhaustible. But there is one important place to start—namely, in medical schools with future health care practitioners.

It is no accident that the rise of bioethics is not just a clinical phenomenon, but an educational one as well. Medical schools have followed the lead of medicine itself by implementing bioethics and humanities classes and programs. Accreditation boards for medical school now demand such offerings for medical students. But the mere existence of a curricula should not be taken as an end in itself. A commitment to teaching medicine as a *social* science concerned with the *human* condition in all aspects of medical education, starting with admissions and ending with continuing education courses, is the ideal; that is what the practice of medicine itself entails.

If this book has argued nothing else, it has attempted to make clear the need to coordinate means and ends. The process of becoming a physician must mirror the kind of physician we wish to produce.[2] Thus, if medical practice is to go beyond mere biochemistry and technological ability, medical curricula must as well, and not merely by developing bioethics and humanities classes marginally, but by making these human concerns integral to the scientific and clinical concerns of the students. We should not expect (particularly in its great complexity) for students to come to medical school as fully developed morally acceptable beings, and we cannot afford to hope that they will spontaneously develop moral habits of medicine once they start practice. Moral artistry is a learned process as much as medical artistry is, and more important, as Edmund Pellegrino has already pointed out, moral artistry is necessary for medical artistry in its fullest sense.

Thus, this book and its arguments and insights are a call to medical education, and other institutions, to reflect on its own methods, to rethink its curricula with an eye not just towards scientific competence but to placing that science into daily operations of social relationships as soon as possible, as often as possible, and as deeply as possible. It is only when our educational habits reflect our concerns and integrate our disciplines for the sake of future ethical medical practice that medicine will fully actualize its potential as an artistically humane *profession*. Physicians will then have at their disposal the habits and tools necessary to profess responsibly their abilities, knowledge, and concern for the human condition as health *care* practitioners.

To generate truly moral encounters, both physicians and patients must be sensitive to the functional possibilities of narrative and meaningful living in the health care community—that is, they must be sensitive, moral artists. And we— the members of our communities, participants in health care, and educators of medical professionals—must facilitate the actualization of these deeper moral possibilities through appropriate means at our disposal that epitomize the morally significant ends that each and every medical encounter can reach, as we both enact and strive for community as healing.

NOTES

1. As was noted in chapter 1, others of my philosophical ilk have already published in bioethics, and should be duly recognized—see, for example, Kegley (1997), Lachs (1995), Mahowald (1993 and 2000), McDermott (1976), McGee (1999 and 2000), Moreno (1995), and Trotter (1997), among others.

2. See note 1 in the previous chapter.

References

Anders, George. 1996. *Health against Wealth: HMOs and the Breakdown of Medical Trust*. New York: Houghton Mifflin.

Annas, George J. 1988. *Judging Medicine*. Clifton, N.J.: Humana.

Beauchamp, Tom L., and James F. Childress. 1979. *Principles of Biomedical Ethics*. New York: Oxford University Press. (See abbreviations section.)

——. 1994. *Principles of Biomedical Ethics*. 4th ed. New York: Oxford University Press. (See abbreviations section.)

Beecher, Henry K. 1966. Ethics and Clinical Research. *New England Journal of Medicine* 74:1354–60.

Bernstein, J. M. 1990. Self-Knowledge as Praxis: Narrative and Narration in Psychoanalysis. In *Narrative in Culture*. Edited by Christopher Nash. New York: Routledge.

Blustein, Jeffrey. 1991. *Care and Commitment: Taking the Personal Point of View*. New York: Oxford University Press.

Buchanan, James H. 1989. *Patient Encounters*. New York: Henry Holt.

Buchler, Justus. 1979. *Toward a General Theory of Human Judgment*. New York: Dover.

Burrell, David, and Stanley Hauerwas. 1979. From System to Story: An Alternative Pattern for Rationality in Ethics. In *Why Narrative? Readings in Narrative Theology*. Edited by Stanley Hauerwas and L. George Jones. Grand Rapids, Mich.: W. B. Eerdmans, 158–90.

Chambers, Tod. 1999. *The Fiction of Bioethics: Cases as Literary Texts*. New York: Routledge.

Clouser, K. Danner, and Bernard Gert. 1990. A Critique of Principlism. *Journal of Medicine and Philosophy* 15:219–36.

DeVries, Raymond, and Peter Conrad. 1998. Why Bioethics Needs Sociology. In *Bioethics and Society: Constructing the Ethical Enterprise*. Edited by Raymond DeVries and Janardan Subedi. Upper Saddle River, N.J.: Prentice Hall, 233–57.

DeVries, Raymond, and Janardan Subedi, eds. 1998. *Bioethics and Society: Constructing the Ethical Enterprise*. Upper Saddle River, N.J.: Prentice Hall.

Dewey, John. 1910. *How We Think*. New York: D. C. Heath. (Also in MW6.)

——. [1916] 1940. *Democracy and Education*. Reprint, New York: Free Press. (Also in MW9.)

———. [1920] 1948. *Reconstruction in Philosophy*. Reprint, Boston: Beacon. (Also in MW12.)

———. [1922] 1930. *Human Nature and Conduct*. Reprint, New York: Modern Library. (Also in MW14.)

———. [1927] 1954. *The Public and Its Problems*. Reprint, Athens, Ohio: Swallow. (Also in LW2.)

———. [1930] 1962. *Individualism, Old and New*. Reprint, New York: Capricorn. (Also in LW5.)

———. 1932. *Ethics*. Rev. ed. With James Tufts. New York: Henry Holt. (Also in LW7.)

———. [1932] 1980. *Theory of the Moral Life*. Edited by Victor Kestenbaum. Reprint, New York: Irvington. (Also in LW7.)

———. [1935] 1963. *Liberalism and Social Action*. Reprint, New York: Capricorn. (Also in LW11.)

———. 1938. *Logic: The Theory of Inquiry*. New York: Henry Holt. (Also in LW12.)

— — —. 1976–1983. *John Dewey: The Middle Works: 1899–1924*. 15 vols. Edited by Jo Ann Boydston. Carbondale: Southern Illinois University Press. (See abbreviations section.)

———. 1981–1990. *John Dewey: The Later Works: 1825–1953*. 17 vols. Edited by Jo Ann Boydston. Carbondale: Southern Illinois University Press. (See abbreviations section.)

Eldridge, Michael. 1996. Dewey's Faith in Democracy as Shared Experience. *Transactions of the Charles S. Peirce Society* 32 (1): 11–30.

Engelhardt Jr., H. Tristram. 1986. *The Foundations of Bioethics*. New York: Oxford University Press. (See abbreviations section.)

———. 1996. *The Foundations of Bioethics*. 2d ed. New York: Oxford University Press. (See abbreviations section.)

Fesmire, Steven A. 1995. Dramatic Rehearsal and the Moral Artist: A Deweyan Theory of Moral Understanding. *Transactions of the Charles S. Peirce Society* 21:568–97.

Fletcher, Joseph. 1954. *Morals and Medicine*. Boston: Beacon.

Flexner, Abraham. 1925. *Medical Education: A Comprehensive Study*. New York: Macmillan.

Frank, Arthur. 1997. Enacting Illness Stories: When, What, and Why. In *Stories and Their Limits: Narrative Approaches to Bioethics*. Edited by Hilde L. Nelson. New York: Routledge, 31–49.

Gert, Bernard. 1988. *Morality: A New Justification of Moral Rules*. New York: Oxford University Press.

Gilligan, Carol. 1993. *In a Different Voice*. Cambridge, Mass.: Harvard University Press.

Hardwig, John. 1997. Autobiography, Biography, and Narrative Ethics. In *Stories and Their Limits: Narrative Approaches to Bioethics*. Edited by Hilde L. Nelson. New York: Routledge, 50–64.

Hester, D. Micah. 1998. The Place of Community in Medical Encounters. *Journal of Medicine and Philosophy* 23 (4): 369–83.

———. 1999. Habits of Healing: Developing Community in Medical Encounters. In *Pragmatic Bioethics*. Edited by Glenn E. McGee. Nashville, Tenn.: Vanderbilt University Press, 45–59.

Inlander, Charles B., et al. 1991. *Take This Book to the Hospital with You*. New York: Wing.

James, William. [1882] 1977. The Sentiment of Rationality. In *The Writings of William James*. Edited by John J. McDermott. Chicago: University of Chicago Press, 317–42.

———. [1890] 1950. *The Principles of Psychology*. 2 vols. Reprint, New York: Dover.

———. [1897] 1956. *The Will to Believe (and Other Essays on Popular Philosophy)*. Reprint, New York: Dover.

———. [1897] 1977. The Moral Philosopher and the Moral Life. In *The Writings of William James*. Edited by John J. McDermott. Chicago: University of Chicago Press, 610–29.

———. [1899a] 1977. On a Certain Blindness in Human Beings. In *The Writings of William James*. Edited by John J. McDermott. Chicago: University of Chicago Press, 629–45.

———. [1899b] 1977. What Makes a Life Significant. In *The Writings of William James*. Edited by John J. McDermott. Chicago: University of Chicago Press, 645–60.

———. [1902] 1958. *The Varieties of Religious Experience*. Reprint, New York: Mentor Books.

———. [1904] 1977. Does "Consciousness" Exist? In *The Writings of William James*. Edited by John J. McDermott. Chicago: University of Chicago Press, 169–83.

———. 1977. *The Writings of William James*. Edited by John J. McDermott. Chicago: University of Chicago Press.

Jones, James H. 1993. *Bad Blood*. 2d ed. New York: Free Press.

Jonsen, Albert. 1997. The Birth of Bioethics: The Origins and Evolution of a Demi-Discipline. *Medical Humanities Review* 11 (1): 9–21.

Jonsen, Albert, and Steven Toulmin. 1988. *The Abuse of Casuistry*. Berkeley: University of California Press.

Jonsen, Albert, Mark Siegler, and William Winslade. 1992. *Clinical Ethics*. 3d ed. New York: McGraw-Hill.

Kant, Immanuel. [1785] 1949. *Critique of Practical Reason (and Other Writings in Moral Philosophy)*. Edited and translated by Lewis White Beck. Reprint, Chicago: University of Chicago Press.

Kegley, Jacquelyn Ann K. 1997. *Genuine Individuals and Genuine Communities*. Nashville, Tenn.: Vanderbilt University Press.

Keith, Heather E. 1997. Pragmatism and Social Ecology: George Herbert Mead's Empathetic Self. Paper presented at meeting of Tennessee Philosophical Association, November 8, 1997, at Vanderbilt University.

Kleinman, Arthur. 1988. *The Illness Narratives*. New York: Basic.

Lachs, John. 1995. *The Relevance of Philosophy to Life*. Nashville, Tenn.: Vanderbilt University Press.

Loewy, Erich. 1997. *Moral Strangers, Moral Acquaintance, and Moral Friends: Connectedness and Its Conditions*. Albany, N.Y.: SUNY Press.

MacIntyre, Alasdair. 1984. *After Virtue*. 2d ed. Notre Dame, Ind.: University of Notre Dame Press.

Mahowald, Mary. 1993. *Women and Children in Health Care: An Unequal Majority*. New York: Oxford University Press.

———. 2000. *Genes, Women, Equity*. New York: Oxford University Press.

McDermott, John J. 1976. Feeling as Insight: The Affective Dimension in Social Diagnosis. In *The Culture of Experience*. Prospect Heights, Ill.: Waveland.

McGee, Glenn E., ed. 1999. *Pragmatic Bioethics*. Nashville, Tenn.: Vanderbilt University Press.

——. 2000. *The Perfect Baby: Parenthood in the New World of Cloning and Genetics*. Lanham, Md.: Rowman & Littlefield.

Mead, George Herbert. [1932] 1980. *The Philosophy of the Present*. Edited by Arthur E. Murphy. Reprint, Chicago: University of Chicago Press.

——. [1934] 1962. *Mind, Self, and Society*. Edited by Charles W. Morris. Reprint, Chicago: University of Chicago Press.

——. [1938] 1972. *The Philosophy of the Act*. Edited by Charles W. Morris. Reprint, Chicago: University of Chicago Press.

——. 1964. *Selected Writings*. Edited by Andrew J. Reck. Chicago: University of Chicago Press.

——. 1982. *The Individual and the Social Self*. Edited by David L. Miller. Chicago: University of Chicago Press.

Moreno, Jonathan D. 1995. *Deciding Together: Bioethics and Moral Consensus*. New York: Oxford University Press.

Morris, Donald. 1996. *Dewey and the Behavioristic Context of Ethics*. Bethesda, Md.: International Scholars.

Munson, Ronald, ed. 2000. *Intervention and Reflection: Basic Issues in Medical Ethics*. 6th ed. Belmont, Calif.: Wadsworth Publishing.

Nagel, Ernest. 1986. Introduction to *John Dewey: The Later Works: 1825–1953*. Vol. 12. Edited by Jo Ann Boydston. Carbondale: Southern Illinois University Press, ix–xxvi.

Nelson, Hilde L., ed. 1997. *Stories and Their Limits: Narrative Approaches to Bioethics*. New York: Routledge.

Novack, Dennis H., et al. 1979. Changes in Physicians' Attitudes toward Telling the Cancer Patient. In *Ethical Issues in Death and Dying*. Edited by Tom Beauchamp and Robert Veatch. Upper Saddle River, N.J.: Prentice Hall, 69–75.

Peirce, Charles Sanders. 1992. *The Essential Peirce*. Vol. 1. Edited by N. Houser and C. Kleosel. Bloomington: Indiana University Press.

——. 1998. *The Essential Peirce*. Vol. 2. Edited by The Peirce Edition Project. Bloomington: Indiana University Press.

Pellegrino, Edmund D. 1979. Anatomy of a Clinical Judgment: Some Notes on Right Reason and Right Action. In *Clinical Judgment: A Critical Appraisal*. Edited by H. Tristram Engelhardt et al. Dordrecht, Holland: D. Reidel Publishing, 169–94.

Pellegrino, Edmund D., and David C. Thomasma. 1993. *The Virtues of Medical Practice*. New York: Oxford University Press.

Pence, Gregory E. 2000. *Classic Cases in Medical Ethics*. 3d ed. New York: McGraw-Hill.

Ramsey, Paul. 1970. *Patient as Person*. New Haven, Conn.: Yale University Press.

Rawls, John. 1971. *A Theory of Justice*. Cambridge, Mass.: Harvard University Press.

Reverby, Susan M., ed. 2000. *Tuskegee's Truths: Rethinking the Tuskegee Syphilis Study*. Chapel Hill: North Carolina University Press.

Rothman, David J. 1991. *Strangers at the Bedside*. New York: Basic.

Royce, Josiah. 1995. *The Philosophy of Loyalty*. Nashville, Tenn.: Vanderbilt University Press.

Sacks, Oliver. 1990. *Awakenings*. New York: Harper Perennial.

——. 1995. *An Anthropologist on Mars*. New York: Knopf.

Schaffner, Kenneth F., ed. 1985. *Logic of Discovery and Diagnosis in Medicine*. Berkeley: University of California Press.

Shelp, Earl E., ed. 1985. *Virtue and Medicine: Explorations in the Character of Medicine*. Dordrecht, Holland: D. Reidel Publishing.

Sigerist, Henry. 1951. *A History of Medicine*. New York: Oxford University Press.

Singer, Beth. 1995. Difference, Otherness, and Creation of Community. Unpublished manuscript received directly from the author.

Sommers, Christina Hoff. 2000. *The War against Boys: How Misguided Feminism Is Harming Our Young Men*. New York: Simon & Schuster.

Strong, Carson. 1997. Is There No Common Morality? *Medical Humanities Review* 11 (1): 39–45.

Talisse, Robert B. 2000. A Critical Study of Liberalism. Ph.D. diss., City University of New York.

Trotter, Griffin. 1997. *The Loyal Physician*. Nashville, Tenn.: Vanderbilt University Press.

Veatch, Robert M. 1981. *A Theory of Medical Ethics*. New York: Basic.

———. 1991. *The Physician–Patient Relationship: The Patient as Partner*, pt 2. Bloomington: Indiana University Press.

White, Kerr L., ed. 1988. *The Task of Medicine*. Menlo Park, Calif.: Henry J. Kaiser Family Foundation.

Wolpe, Paul Root. 1998. The Triumph of Autonomy in American Bioethics: A Sociological View. In *Bioethics and Society: Constructing the Ethical Enterprise*. Edited by Raymond DeVries and Janardan Subedi. Upper Saddle River, N.J.: Prentice Hall, 38–59.

Zaner, Richard M. 1988. *Ethics and the Clinical Encounter*. Upper Saddle River, N.J.: Prentice Hall.

———. 1993. *Troubled Voices*. Cleveland: Pilgrim's Press.

Index

ability (abilities), 62, 66n19, 70, 72, 85;
    critical, 10; to fit stories together, 58;
    rational, 35; technical, 59, 76, 80, 85
act(s), 16, 26, 35, 50, 55; deceptive,
    38n10; meaningful, 67; paternalistic,
    75–76
action(s), 6–7, 9, 11–13, 15, 16, 24–27,
    30, 33–34, 40–43, 45, 49, 51–52, 57,
    60, 62, 65n7, 67, 71; autonomous,
    40–41; determined, 36–37; enlightened
    paternalistic, 77; guidelines for, 22;
    moral, 30; right healing, 5–6, 17
activity (activities), 7–8, 10–11, 14,
    16–17, 23–24, 26, 29, 34, 44, 49,
    51–52, 55, 68, 70, 71–73, 76;
    biochemical, 48; constructive, 44;
    courageous, 63; ethical, 33, 35–36, 39;
    habit-developed, 8; imaginative, 12;
    intelligent, 7, 12, 33; as meaningful,
    61, 66n19; as mechanical and artificial,
    16; moral, 12–14, 25, 31, 40–42, 45,
    51; regulating and adjusting, 52;
    sharing of, 52, 64n6; social, 71
adjustment(s), 7–8, 24, 65n6; reflective, 24
affections, 71–72
affliction(s), 68, 73
agency, 47; patient, 40, 68, 74–75
agent(s), 1, 56; autonomous, 41–42, 44;
    moral, 38n14, 40
agreement: as constitutive of moral
    communities, 32; mutual, 30

AIDS, 11
ailment(s), 69–71, 75
ALS. *See* amyotrophic lateral sclerosis
Alzheimer's disease, 22, 40
American Association of Medical
    Colleges, 18n1
amputation, 36–37
amyotrophic lateral sclerosis, 74, 78
anatomy, 61; anatomical structures, 56
argument(s), 30, 36, 37, 53, 77; of this
    book, 83–85; rational, 29–30, 43
art, 6
asymetry in medicine. *See*
    physician–patient relationship,
    asymmetrical
attitude(s), 10–11, 48, 77; acceptable,
    81n6; community (communities),
    49–50, 54, 56; incoherence with
    experiences, 44; liberal, 59; of others,
    49–51; personal, 59, 80; prevailing, 76;
    shared, 51; unique nexus of social, 54
authority: in action, 42; final, 29; moral,
    29–31
authorship: problem of, 58
autonomous: by degrees, 40; requirement
    that an action be substantially, 41;
    sufficiently, 41
autonomy, 3, 14–16, 18, 31, 40–42, 44,
    46–47, 56, 64, 76–77, 84; as absence
    of coercive influences, 3; alternative to,
    47; as consent, 81n10; Enlightenment,

About the Author

D. Micah Hester is assistant professor of biomedical ethics and humanities at Mercer University's School of Medicine in Macon, Georgia. He received his Ph.D. in philosophy from Vanderbilt University, where he specialized in bioethics and American philosophy. In addition to this book, Hester has also written journal articles and book chapters in bioethics and has coauthored or coedited six books in American philosophy, computer ethics, and the philosophy of education. Presently, he is researching the subject of end-of-life care for a manuscript for future publication.